*Time Out
for
Motherhood*

Time Out

for

Motherhood

A Guide for Today's Working Woman

to the Financial, Emotional, and

Career Aspects of Having a Baby

Lucy Scott, Ph.D., and
Meredith Joan Angwin

JEREMY P. TARCHER, INC. Los Angeles
Distributed by St. Martin's Press New York

Library of Congress Cataloging-in-Publication Data

Scott, Lucy, 1928–
  Time out for motherhood.

  Bibliography: p.
  Includes index.
  1. Working mothers—United States.   2. Childbirth
in middle age—United States.   3. Motherhood—Economic
aspects—United States.   4. Choice (Psychology)
I. Angwin, Meredith.   II. Title.
HQ759.48.S36   1986   306.8′743   86-3732
ISBN 0-87477-382-2

Jeremy P. Tarcher, Inc.
9110 Sunset Blvd.
Los Angeles, CA 90069

Design by Jane A. Thurmond

Manufactured in the United States of America
10 9 8 7 6 5 4 3 2 1

First Edition

To our parents
Amos and Fern Hoff,
and Beatrice Stein Light

and our children
Cynthia, Susan, Julia, and Ilan

C O N T E N T S

During approximately the past decade, the industrialized nations of the world have noted a trend toward later motherhood. Many women are having their first child at an age when a quarter of a century ago most families were complete.

During a decade as a practicing pediatrician and as a member of the board of directors of an innovative child-care program, I have found very little published with these mothers in mind. *Time Out for Motherhood* is especially pertinent to the new, but older, mother. It is a remarkably inclusive book that can be read in its entirety before the prospective mother embarks on motherhood, and can also be referred to as a guide during and after pregnancy. Some sections are almost unique in child-care literature, especially the chapter on budgetary matters and financial planning for a baby.

With the skills and resources a woman has acquired while delaying motherhood, and the assistance of a guide such as this one, later motherhood may indeed be better.

Frederick A. Lloyd, M.D., F.A.A.P.
Clinical Professor of Pediatrics
Stanford University School of Medicine

Member, Board of Directors
Palo Alto Community Child Care

(Editor's note: Palo Alto Community Child Care (PACCC) runs ten day-care centers, serving a total of 300 children.

It also runs a "recuperating child service" for its infant-toddler program, and maintains an alliance with a day-care mothers' network. It is also active in informing parents of day-care issues and options. PACCC is partially funded by the City of Palo Alto.)

The creation of this book began long before we two met. It began with our emotional commitment to a life where there is time for both mothering and working. A life where there is a possibility of taking some time out for motherhood without dropping out of the work world forever.

Both of us have combined careers and mothering. Lucy Scott obtained her Ph.D. and began her teaching and counseling career after her daughters were born. Her doctoral research focused on women who chose to be parents later in their lives. For five years, she headed the Parenthood After Thirty Project, a resource center for women making the parenthood decision. Currently, she is supervisor of Parents Place, in San Francisco, a model resource and referral agency for parents. Meredith Angwin first got her master's degree in physical chemistry and then had children. For Meredith, working most of her life as a scientist has constituted its own learning process, teaching her a great deal about what it means to be a woman who really wants to work and also really wants to raise decent children.

Our book is not meant to be a scientific "review of the literature," but rather to offer advice to a particular group of women moving together through this period in history. Of course, each woman makes her own choice about motherhood, shaped by her own unique situation; but these unique situations are necessarily shaped by the context in which we find ourselves, the world of the '80s. The world of the double image, the woman executive and the nurturing mother—a balance achievable only in a day that has more than twenty-four hours. In writing this book we have relied mainly on our common sense and our own experience as mothers to evaluate the psychological research. We have concluded that women can indeed have it all— a productive career and children, too—if they are willing to have realistic expectations of themselves. And realistic expectations include taking at least a few months off for each baby.

This book is not about how to be superwoman. If you think that all problems can be solved by time management, then you should probably buy a different book (*The One-Minute Mother*?). Better yet, buy this one, and get a feeling for what time is: Time is your life. A child will bring drastic changes to every facet of your life: your relationships, your job, and your finances. Be willing to grow, change, and mature with your new role.

Which brings us to finances. One reason that women delay having a child is the rational fear that they cannot afford one. We therefore felt that a chapter on financial planning was absolutely essential. Underlying this chapter, however, is a philosophy, which comes down to the fact that ultimately finances are in your control. While older parents are often more financially secure than younger people, they are also more realistic. So they worry more. We hope that our financial planning sections will both alleviate anxiety and provide useful advice for planning for a child.

And now it is time to thank people. Until we wrote the book, Meredith often wondered how the acknowledgment lists in books got so long. Well, now she knows.

First, we would like to thank our families, for inspiring us and encouraging us to write the book, as well as for being kind to us while we wrote it. Lucy is especially grateful to her two daughters, Cynthia and Susan, who continually urged her to "put into print what you know." Meredith would like to thank her husband, George, for his unfailing trust and encouragement. And she would like to thank her supervisor at the Electric Power Research Institute, J. Peter N. Paine, for his forbearance. All these people will have many reasons to be glad to see the book in print (finally!).

And without Janice Gallagher, our editor ("Some nice thoughts here—let me give you some ideas for organizing them"), it would not be the book it is. Thank you, Janice, for your good advice.

Other people who gave us good advice include Dr. Howard Blanchette, M.D., who reviewed the chapter on older pregnancy, and Dr. Frederick Lloyd, M.D., who reviewed the chapters on the new baby and on day care. We are also indebted to Professor Shirley Feldman of Stanford and Professor Eleanor Willemsen of the University of Santa Clara for discussions on the psychological consequences of being an older mother, as well as on day care. Also, a special thank you to Marty Sochet, a leader in fatherhood seminars, and to Debby Lee, of the Early Single Parenting Project, for their advice on the fatherhood and single motherhood chapters. Any errors in the book, however, are our own, and not the responsibility of our reviewers.

Several people read and commented upon the various parts of the manuscript. We appreciate their feedback and their time. In alphabetical order, they are Bill Abbott, George Angwin, Jennifer and Tom Arnold, Lee Bonds, Carole Girvan, Ulla Gustafsson, Carolyn MacHale, Debby MacIntosh, Susan McCarthy, Betsy Roeth, Lori Twersky, Tom York, and Alan and Cathy Zimmerman. Also, thanks to Jacky Hood for the timely loan of a letter-quality printer.

Finally, we would like to thank the many people we interviewed and the men and women who shared their questions and concerns with Lucy at her decision-making workshops and in her clinical practice. Your names are not here, to protect your privacy, but your insights and concerns are a vital part of the book.

Time Out

for

Motherhood

Making the Motherhood Decision

Having a Baby—
Now

Seven years. That is the average length of time between a woman's graduation from college and the magic age of thirty, when she becomes "old." Or at least, when she becomes an "older mother," a "special problem" if she "delayed" having children during those seven years.

The time available for starting a family is even more limited for women who go on to medical, graduate, or professional school. Having a baby while you are a full-time student is usually impractical. Having a baby the moment you graduate, before even working in your field, seems genuinely wasteful.

College graduates or not, most women are in the work force for the majority of their lives. And that means that getting an education and/or a start on work is their major goal while they are in their twenties. The modern twenty-year-old woman is likely to become an older mother simply because there just isn't time enough in that decade to do everything.

Today's older mothers comprise the first generation of women who had access to the birth control pill and to legal abortion. The women's movement had direct influence on their hopes and self-expectations. Their life goals call for an extensive preparental agenda: education, career, and most of all, maturity.

The proportion of childless women in their twenties doubled during the early '70s. In the following decade, the rate of first births for women between thirty and thirty-four more than tripled, the largest increase in birth rate of any age group.

Most of today's women are not interested in going from the classroom to the diaper pail without having some time to achieve a certain amount of self-knowledge. The phrase "giving birth to myself before I give birth to a baby" is one that more and more women are using to describe their approach to having children.

Educated modern women are rejecting the "seven-year window" as the only time in which to start a family and instead are beginning to follow their own agendas. They are having babies when they feel emotionally and financially ready to do so.

Similar shifts are taking place in the institution of marriage. Twenty years ago, a woman usually expected to be married by age twenty-two, at which time she would risk becoming an old maid. As one woman said, "I remember this feeling of complete panic when I realized that graduation was approaching and I wasn't engaged. My friends were engaged, and my parents certainly expected it." The marriage time-schedule is no longer so rigid—and neither is the baby schedule.

Nonetheless, books about older motherhood usually concentrate on the perceived problems: infertility, birth defects, long labors. They ignore the fact that these problems are rare (except for infertility, which has been described by some doctors as a national epidemic). Most women of any age who get pregnant will have healthy children. And psychologically, older is often better.

YOU'RE NOT AN OLDER MOTHER, YOU'RE A BETTER MOTHER

The younger woman, who has her babies at the "right" time, belongs to the traditional majority of women who give birth to their first and last child in their twenties. But though tradition is on her side, her attitude often leaves something to be desired. She may feel that the baby is interrupting her life, her ability to establish herself as her own person. She often sees her child as the "reason" she can't take trips, get a good job, or go back to school. She may be postponing independence, achievement, and self-knowledge.

The thirty-year-old mother has a different set of considerations. She usually doesn't need any excuses for where she is with her life, and her love, patience, and readiness can ultimately develop an excellent rapport with her baby. Dr. Shirley Feldman, a psychologist at Stanford University, studies age-related parenting issues. Describing older mothers, she says: "It's readiness. The older mother just seems to do better with the infant with every test we've devised."

Other studies also show the older mother as doing very well. The children of older mothers tend to do better in school and on IQ tests. The mothers themselves are economically ahead of women who had their children earlier.

Let's look at the children's development first. Several investigators have studied the correlation between maternal age and children's IQ. The effect of maternal age is small, but it is positive and persistent. As Arlene Ragozin of the University of Washington noted in a paper, the good effect of increased maternal age can be seen when examining the entire child-bearing age range—that is, in studies focusing on mothers of different ages, older motherhood was correlated with children having higher IQs and also higher school achievement.

Why do the children of older mothers test out brighter? Is it hereditary (the implication being that people who wait are smart)? Actually, it is probably environment. Older mothers tend to do a better job of interacting with their babies, and seem to enjoy motherhood more.

Dr. Feldman and her students at Stanford observed mother-infant interactions through one-way mirrors. They counted "suitable interactions" between mothers and babies—mothers cooing at or playing with the baby, for example. In these tests, being an older mother was correlated with being a better mother.

In a similar study, Arlene Ragozin also observed mothers and babies through one-way mirrors. Here the mothers were asked to imitate the babies, in order to determine how sensitive the mothers were to the babies own cues. First-time older mothers did best in these tests. All second-time mothers did about the same, and older mothers with a third child did somewhat worse than younger mothers.

Another part of these studies focused on discussions with the mothers, not simply observation of them. Older first-time mothers were happiest with their roles and most satisified with their baby's development.

No other factors besides age were as good a predictor of appropriate mother-baby interactions. Some of the families in the Ragozin study, for example, were middle-class, while others were on welfare (the researchers called this "public or private sources of income"). This crude measure of socioeconomic status could not predict good mothering. Age of the mother was still the best predictor.

Having a baby at a nontraditional time also makes good economic sense. This is clear from talking to women ("I wanted to get my M.B.A. first," or, "I wanted to get established in my job before taking time out") and is borne out by the limited amount of research that has been done on economics and age of parenting.

At the Center for Population Research in Washington, Sandra Hoffreth did a study, "Long-Term Economic Consequences for Women of Delayed Childbearing and Reduced Family Size," in which the women studied were sixty and older. Her results: "Women who delay a first birth [past thirty] have higher family incomes and living standards . . . [and] appear to be able to accumulate greater assets than those who bear their children at an average age."

Hoffreth's results offer small, tantalizing, but ultimately unsatisfying tidbits of information. Why did the women delay their children's births? Because they married later? Because they were ambitious in their jobs? The results don't answer these questions; they just provide more pieces to the puzzle.

Nevertheless, the entire scope of the answer is becoming clear. A woman over thirty who becomes a mother is not a "special problem." She is more likely to be a good example: good with her child, economically secure, emotionally ready for motherhood.

While older mothers are better mothers, the choice to become an older mother is rarely easy. As one gets older, life gets more complicated. Financial obligations, career involvement, commitments to husbands, friends, and hobbies—all these begin to seem fixed and immovable. The underlying concern of most women who are considering pregnancy in their thirties is how to fit their life together with a baby added in. *How can I make it all work?*

The first part of this book provides information to help in the to-have-or-not-to-have-a-baby decision. Offered are facts about the medical risks—what the problems are, what can you do to increase your (already very good) chances of having a healthy baby, the costs of child-rearing, and suggestions for financial planning.

But since child-bearing decisions are not made simply on the basis of facts and figures, we also consider the important relationships in a woman's life: the potential father, or the support structures for women who will be single mothers. This section ends with a chapter on actually making the decision: putting the facts and feelings together and resolving the question: Is motherhood for me?

The second half of the book, "Pregnancy and Beyond," describes fitting a child into your life. It discusses the experience of pregnancy, the stress of the first months (and how to alleviate it), and decisions on work and day care. It offers practical advice for women who are going to be mothers in their thirties. But there is no law against reading the second half of the book before you make your decision. It will help you understand what having a child in your life will actually mean.

We have met too many over-thirty mothers and mothers-to-be to believe that they would be satisfied with a book that details every medical risk of later pregnancy and then drops the subject at the delivery table—as if, once the older mother has given birth to a healthy baby, her problems are over. Or at least, that her problems are no different than those of a twenty-year-old new mother, who has no investment in a job and no mortgage on a house. We believe that older mothers, women who are deeply involved in many facets of life besides motherhood when they choose to have a baby, deserve a book that recognizes this fact. The goal here is to help the mother in all phases of her informed choice.

The first step toward this informed choice is to shake free of the myths perpetrated throughout society, myths about women who bake chocolate-chip cookies every day as after-school treats and have children without cavities. Myths about women on the fast track up the corporate ladder, who give birth in between other exciting assignments. Only by examining these images and seeing through these tales can we begin to see reality.

DOUBLE IMAGE

The question *How can I decide about having a baby?* can be rephrased: *How can I resolve two competing sets of images—the working woman and the mother?* The availability of gray flannel suits on maternity racks does not really answer this concern.

Reliable birth control and the women's movement brought a splendid new world into women's reach—a world of career choices unhampered by unwanted pregnancies, a world where it is possible to do a man's job and perhaps even earn a man's salary. A world of the New Woman. Without frequent pregnancies, a marriage could be more of an equal partnership and less of an economic dependency. The world of work could yield its joys: financial independence, the recognition of co-workers, seeing a project through from idea to accomplishment, perhaps travel. For many women in their late twenties and thirties, however, the image of the New Woman in this world has its dark side. The biological clock is ticking, and the price for putting motherhood on hold increases.

Another image comes to mind here, an older picture: woman as mother. These are the ancient images: little, fat fertility goddesses, almost the first artifacts humans made when they got beyond the flint-chipping stage. The woman as Mother has been loved, she has been worshipped—the Madonna and Child, the Egyptian mother-goddess Isis with infant Horus at her breast. And perhaps there are memories of one's own childhood: rocking chairs, cookies and milk, warmth, safety, security, a selfless nurturer.

So while there may be a New Woman in the world, where is the New Mother? There is possibly a concept of the Working Mother, but that brings to mind neglected children, meetings cut short because the day-care center closes at 5:30, and a harried life, short on time and long on compromises. The ultimate ideal of the mother has not changed from ancient times. She is young, nurturing, soft, and absorbed in her love for her children, who form the center of her life.

The real modern woman is caught between images— between the woman that plays the rough corporate games mother never taught her and the woman who *is* mother, amusing her child with this-little-piggie games that can't hurt.

Dress for success or wear clothes that make it easy to nurse a baby? Career or motherhood? The childless woman of thirty-one or thirty-two is most vulnerable to distress from these unresolved images. She has invested a lot in her job, in her relative economic independence. She has tasted satisfactions of the work world and is also familiar with the strain. Her expectations of herself have grown with her confidence. "I know that if I had children, I could be a perfect mother," says a lawyer in her early thirties, discussing her ambivalence about having children. Her ideal of motherhood (and she doesn't want to do it unless she can do it *right*) includes nursing the babies, teaching the preschoolers herself, and being involved with the children's school and the PTA. But she is unsure: How can she take on the job of perfect motherhood and still be a lawyer?

Motherhood involves giving up total control of one's body and one's life. It means putting up with the discomforts and restrictions of pregnancy for the sake of the baby. It means giving up a hard-won sense of mastery and entering a situation of truly awe-inspiring unpredictability. Giving up control can feel like a step backward.

But choosing against motherhood doesn't feel right, either. Certainly, society is now more understanding of women who choose not to have children, but for every woman who really has known all along that she didn't want children there are a hundred who always expected to be mothers "someday." For a childless woman in her thirties, "someday" has suddenly turned into "now."

It doesn't look as if help with this decision will come from the women's movement. The movement doesn't seem to discuss motherhood very much. *Ms. Magazine* offers "Stories for Free Children" about nonsexist child-raising. There is some attention to government policies and support for day care. Endless statistics are presented on female-headed households and employment equity. On the other hand, there is very little discussion of women's requirements for a balance of love and work in their lives.

This is because most of the attention has been focused on economic inequities between men and women in the job market—scrutiny that has not been wasted. More women than ever are mayors, lawyers, engineers, unionized blue-collar workers. But the central issue of modern motherhood remains unresolved. Balance between love and work is different for a woman. For a man, becoming a father has psychological implications, but usually no direct career consequences. For a woman, motherhood brings profound changes—in her body, her emotions, and usually in her attitude toward her career. Once a woman is a mother, whether to work or how many hours to work (part-time? full-time? seventy hours a week?) is more than a financial or career decision. It becomes a matter of goals and balance.

The women's movement as a whole has shown little interest in how to achieve this balance, although as its leaders have personally grown older they have begun to address the question.

When Betty Friedan discussed love and nurturing in her book *The Second Stage,* she was roundly denounced by more militant women for giving up her feminist principles. But Friedan felt it important to note that the issues facing modern women go far beyond those currently addressed by feminism. It does not come down simply to equal pay; there are real questions beyond the paycheck. Is there a portion of a woman's life that can or should be spent in the endeavors unique to women: bearing a child, nursing it, raising toddlers?

Friedan noted that she was essentially a housewife while she was working on *The Feminine Mystique.* She quit writing each day when her daughter came home from school. She took her freedom to take care of her children for granted, while she wrote the book that pointed out that a lifetime as a wife and mother is not satisfactory. Now she talks to women who have succeeded on the job but have never felt they had the freedom to be mothers: "I fought so hard to get here, but after all, once I made it—really— it's just a job."

Germaine Greer, in *Sex and Destiny,* stated the matter even more forcefully: "White western women have given up their only true destiny: motherhood. Duped into futile competition with men, they have come to hate children and fear their own fertility." This book was published when Greer was forty-six and childless.

As Friedan wrote in *The Feminine Mystique*, motherhood as a career was not the answer. But a career instead of motherhood is not the answer either, at least not for most women. Older mothers have the advantage of combining career and motherhood, but for a woman in her twenties, work versus motherhood often is (and feels) like an either-or-decision. Older women tend to have the maturity to combine their roles, since they are generally more secure in their jobs and can often obtain lengthy maternity leaves from employers who would replace a younger or less experienced woman. Moreover, the older a woman is, the more she is likely to earn. This removes some constraints from her child-care decision; she doesn't have to put up with inadequate care just because it is inexpensive. She is more likely to have the maturity to make good decisions and arrangements, along with the skill to carry out her plans.

But why does it take so much skill to arrange for both motherhood and a productive life? Part of the problem is resolving the double image, but another part can be found only by reviewing the economic situation of the '80s.

THE NEW ECONOMIC CONSTRAINTS ON MOTHERHOOD

While employment is often a source of satisfaction and opportunity for personal growth, there are very few women who expect merely self-fulfillment from their jobs; most need a paycheck as well. Many women over thirty consider themselves self-supporting, whether they are married or not.

Economic expectations of women, as well as the overall economic situation, have changed greatly since the 1950s, the decade of the baby boom. Since then, there has been a revolution in more than just women's career expectations; there has also been constant (and sometimes spectacular) inflation. This inflation has affected every aspect of daily life, especially the price and affordability of houses.

Says one woman in California, "My house was built in the '50s. But there is a big difference between the woman who first owned it and myself. She could stay home with her children, whereas I have to work or we couldn't pay the mortgage. I think women like me are just running harder to stay in the same place."

Most of this woman's running in place is due to inflation and high interest rates. In most cities, a middle-class lifestyle has moved beyond the reach of ordinary single-income families.

In the '50s, a man might boast, "I support the family; my wife provides the savings and vacations." Such a statement would seem sexist today, and such a setup would most likely be impractical. But families that count on both incomes in order to meet their living expenses face another sort of problem. Under these circumstances, it is very difficult for a woman to take time out for motherhood.

Most women cannot afford to drop out of the work world to become mothers. And most women who become older mothers do not plan such a retirement. The real problem is whether or not you can interrupt your work participation for a few months or a year.

We discuss financial planning as a solution to this dilemma in the third chapter. With some planning, most older women can take some time off after the baby is born. Even if the woman does not choose to take time off, she will need to plan in order to have enough money to make an appropriate choice of child care. Adequate child care for an infant is expensive; you cannot simply look for the cheapest baby-sitting available (Chapter 10 discusses choosing child care).

In the '50s, during the baby boom, a woman's choice to take time off work for child-raising was less difficult, often because the choice was made for her. For one thing, many companies fired a woman once she got pregnant. And having lost her job, her condition of unemployment was somehow less a burden on her family then than now.

Remember, this was a time when a bank arranging a home mortgage counted only the husband's income in calculating what the family could afford. The wife's income was considered to be infinitely interruptible by child-rearing responsibilities.

Today such employment discrimination against pregnant women is against the law. Bankers are also legally required to consider the wife's income along with the husband's in calculating home loans. Where the '50s banker presumed that all women would be mothers, the '80s banker must assume that no women will be mothers. Or at least that no women will interrupt their earnings significantly in order to be mothers. The banker's new assumptions have allowed the average family to qualify for a much bigger home loan—not necessarily an advantage when it comes to deciding to have children.

Few women want to go back to the days when most men would refuse to "let" their wives work and when women were often summarily dismissed from employment when they got pregnant. But the new order, in which women don't feel they have the option to quit work for a year (or even a few months) for each child, is hardly more satisfying.

It is, however, a situation typical of the inflation-maimed economy that is our heritage in the '80s. Many women reproach themselves (*Why can't I figure out how to afford to have a baby? My parents had me when they weren't particularly rich.*) when the failure is in society. It isn't easy, nowadays, to afford to have a baby. And it isn't easy to choose to have a baby when you aren't sure how you will afford it.

THE PROCESS OF CHOICE

Choice involves information, as well as self-understanding. Mere information is insufficient: What does it matter how much a baby costs if you honestly don't want the burden of raising one? And once you do decide you want to raise a healthy child, then you are obligated to learn how to take care of yourself during pregnancy and how to safeguard a baby's health after birth. (Chapters 2 and 7 discuss pregnancy, and Chapters 8 and 10 are concerned with infant care, including choosing day care.)

Remember that parenthood is a great adventure; and as we all know from the adventurous tales we read as children, adventures are full of the unexpected and the unpredictable. Understanding how much control you can reasonably expect to have is the first step.

For example, you can lower the chances of having a low-birth-weight baby by giving up smoking. But you cannot *guarantee* that you will not have a low-birth-weight baby by *any* method. You can only coax the odds into being in your favor. In pregnancy, control goes only so far.

On the other hand, you probably have more control over your financial life than you may think. Over and over, we have met women who "managed" to take six months off or work part-time, simply by doing a little planning. And even if finances get tight, there aren't any debtor's prisons anymore. Also, many bosses will grant extended part-time leaves to valued employees. As one mother said, "I pushed the system, and I took four months off full-time and the rest of the first year off part-time. My recommendation to any pregnant women is to bargain, to negotiate. Bargain with your boss, bargain with your creditors, if you need to. Time with the baby is worth it, and you never know what you can get until you try."

The decision to have a baby is only the first of a series of choices, for women who combine work with motherhood. To make these choices, you need to thoroughly understand your economic circumstances, as well as your health insurance options. You need to understand what kind of care a baby needs so that you can provide it, either personally or through another source.

Society, with its double image, encourages only two choices: motherhood as a career or motherhood as a six-week "disability" leave to recover from childbirth. We do not believe that either choice is adequate. Motherhood as a career cannot meet the emotional and financial needs of most women; motherhood as a six-week interruption of business-as-usual rarely meets the emotional needs of babies or mothers. Which is why we called our book *Time Out for Motherhood.*

Because we believe in time out. We believe in pushing the system a bit, so that you can spend a few months with your baby. But we don't believe that motherhood ought to cause a retirement from the usual pursuits of adults and a semipermanent retreat to the home. We also don't believe that a woman should enter motherhood without some idea of what effect it will have on her relationship with her husband or on their finances. Raising a child is an activity of the head (making informed choices) as well as of the heart.

The material in this book is designed to help women make informed choices. The information itself is as accurate as possible, but we do not claim that the presentation is unbiased. We are biased. We are in favor of older mothers. We believe that women in their thirties make very good mothers, and that the more information they have the better mothers they are likely to be.

But let us start at the beginning. When Lucy Scott gives workshops as part of her "Parenthood After Thirty" project, one question arises over and over: "I'm over thirty. What are the risks if I get pregnant now? *Can* I have a healthy child?"

Can I Have a Healthy Child? The Medical Concerns of Being an Older Mother

When should a woman have a child? That is a difficult question. When can a woman have a child? That's an easier question, and maybe a better place to start.

Technically, the possibility of pregnancy exists from menarche to menopause, or from the early teens to (possibly) the early fifties. Bearing a healthy child is not guaranteed at any age. Risks are highest for the children of teenage pregnancies and lower for those born when the mother is in her twenties; they creep up again when the mother enters her thirties. The age of thirty-five is considered a boundary line. At this time a woman supposedly enters the high-risk group of the "elderly primagravida," the not-so-flattering technical medical term for a woman having her first pregnancy over thirty-five.

The National Institute of Health finds that women who delay the birth of their first child until the ages of thirty to thirty-four have only a slightly higher chance of problems than younger women do. It is helpful to think of risk as a J-shaped curve, somewhat higher in adolescence, lowest in the twenties, and rising again in the thirties.

However, being thirty-five in itself does not carry with it any biological significance. Some risks increase in the mid-thirties, and age thirty-five is used as a statistical demarcation. But biology is continuous, while statistics are a man-made artifact. There is no "magic date" when it suddenly becomes unsafe to have a baby.

For all prospective mothers of any age, bearing a healthy child is the overriding concern. There are some risks associated with being an older mother, but it takes some statistical skill to assess them. Every pregnancy has its own set of risk factors; the mother's age is simply one among many.

Birth defects are caused by a variety of factors: genetics, the mother's and father's age, the mother's consumption of alcohol, whether or not she smokes, and her general health.

Most birth defects are not related specifically to age. If they were, all a doctor would have to do would be to ask a woman how old she was; then all important risks would be known. Actually, in order to determine risk, the doctor must perform a medical examination and take a thorough medical history.

The doctor will ask about

- the family's genetic and health problems
- the woman's own health history
- her exposure to alcohol, smoking, and drugs
- the current state of her health, weight, and diet
- any occupational hazards she has been exposed to— x-rays, chemicals, radiation, radar
- occupational hazards that the husband may have been exposed to.

The risks for all pregnancies have been decreasing over the years, as medical science and health practices improve. For example, the introduction of immunoglobulin shots (Rhogam) have cut the risks for children of Rh-negative mothers. Better care for premature infants has saved vast numbers of children. Operations for heart defects have been improved; open-heart surgery for some infant heart-defects is now almost standard, while it was experimental and rare twenty years ago. Even considering age-related risks, the risks today for the child of a healthy older mother are just about the same as the risks were for children of all mothers twenty years ago.

However, in one regard the younger mother is definitely at an advantage. Infertility does increase with age, and women over thirty should be aware of this potential problem.

INFERTILITY AND AGE

The first step to motherhood is getting pregnant. Even for women who adopt, the first step toward adoption is usually attempting to get pregnant. Unfortunately, many experts feel that there is an epidemic of infertility now and that the simple equation, "intercourse equals pregnancy," is no longer the assumed certainty it was. Estimates of infertility or fertility impairment range from 15 percent to 20 percent of couples, overall.

It is a common belief that the inability to bear a child is often a sign of neurosis or innate selfishness. But the fact is, most infertility problems are caused by physiological malfunctioning. Since the problem is usually physical, the corrective measures are medical, not psychological. Infertility is no reflection on a couple's worth as human beings, their emotional stability, or their desire to have a child.

The most likely factors to decrease fertility are low sperm-count, blockage of the fallopian tubes, and hormonal imbalance. Other problems that might decrease fertility include fibroid tumors (benign tumors in the uterus) and endometriosis (a condition in which tissue resembling the uterine lining grows elsewhere in the pelvic cavity) in women, and prostate troubles in men. There's also a slightly higher miscarriage and stillbirth rate for older mothers.

Are these age-related problems? Yes and no. Any of these conditions can occur at any age, but the chances of complications increase as one gets older. For example, the chance of having an infection that causes fallopian tube damage tends to increase with age; the woman has simply lived long enough to have heightened the possibility of getting such an infection. The same is true of men and exposure to toxic chemicals: The longer the man has lived, the more likely he is to be exposed to such materials. Other conditions are more simply age-related; for instance, fibroid tumors are more common in older women. Princeton demographers Jane Menkin and Ulla Larsen estimate that 6 percent of women are unable to conceive at ages twenty to twenty-four; 9 percent at twenty-five to twenty-nine; 15 percent at thirty to thirty-four; 30 percent at thirty-five to thirty-nine; and 64 percent at forty to forty-nine.

Nevertheless, there is some good news about infertility. Many infertility problems can now be solved. The solutions comprise such simple measures as reducing excessive exercise, bringing weight into the normal range, or timing intercourse for peak fertile periods. More elaborate methods include drugs and surgery. Most doctors recommend that older couples come in for tests after only six months without conception.

Further reading on infertility can be found in books recommended in the reference section and through the organization Resolve (P.O. Box 474, Belmont, MA 02178). But fear of being infertile should not stop an older woman from attempting to have a child. Even the figure of 30 percent infertility after age thirty-five means that 70 percent of women at that age will have no trouble conceiving.

BEARING A HEALTHY CHILD

The next concern, after conception, is bearing a healthy child. Of course, there is no such thing as a risk-free pregnancy. Various factors affect the degree of risk: the woman's age, health, family history, socioeconomic status, weight, her and her husband's job histories, and quality of medical care. Overall, no woman of any age is guaranteed a healthy baby when she gets pregnant. On the other hand, the converse of that statement is also true: Most women of any age will have healthy babies.

Age-related variables are best known and, to a certain extent, best publicized. For one thing, the age of the mother is known at the child's birth. It is more difficult to determine her occupational history, eating and smoking habits, and family history. Among the variables of most interest to older women are chromosomal abnormalities, although other major defects (which are not strongly age-related) are actually more common.

Genetic Abnormalities: How They Happen and to Whom

From the two-celled beginning of egg and sperm, a baby ultimately results: a baby with eyes, fingernails, hair, inborn responses, a tongue and palate to suck a nipple, and all the other wonders of life. In so complex a growth process, things can go wrong. It is estimated that one out of sixteen babies has a birth defect of some kind, most of them minor: skin discolorations known as birthmarks, or an extra flap of skin on the ear. Major problems can occur at one of two times in the prenatal process: during genetic encoding, or during fetal development. Most defects of either type are evident at birth, though some (such as deafness or learning problems) do not appear for weeks, months, or even years.

The first level of concern is genetic encoding. Chromosomes may carry codes that lead to hereditary diseases, such as Huntington's chorea or Tay-Sachs disease. These are both hereditary, fatal nervous-system diseases. Huntington's chorea strikes its victims in mid-life, while babies born with Tay-Sachs seldom live longer than three years.

In these situations, the father and/or mother is usually a carrier of the gene in question. For example, in sickle cell anemia, common in black people, and thalassemia, a related disease common in people from the Mediterranean region, both father and mother carry a recessive gene, which has little or no effect on their own health. But one-fourth of their children will inherit a double dose of this recessive gene. These children's bodies will make an inadequate form of hemoglobin, which carries oxygen through the blood to the cells of the body, and they will be victims of a debilitating and life-shortening disease.

Carrier couples have truly high-risk pregnancies. They have one chance out of four of bearing a child who will not live to adulthood. They also carry a 50 percent probability of having a child who will inherit the same dangerous recessive gene—a child whose own health will be unaffected, but who will be a carrier himself.

Reviewing risks of this magnitude, the geneticist Theodosius Dobhzhanksy practically despaired of the future of the human race. He foresaw a world in which more and more of society's resources would be devoted to keeping alive the bearers of lethal or debilitating genes. Actually, this is an unlikely scenario. Medical advances hold out to us the hope that one day carrier couples will be easily identified. These couples, once apprised of the risk, may or may not choose to have children. Moreover, there may come a time when these diseases are cured.

Genetic problems of the type described above are no respecters of age. A woman's genetic makeup is in every cell of her body at birth, and it doesn't change as she gets older.

The only major genetic defect for which age makes a difference is Down's syndrome. A child with Down's syndrome has a particular set of facial abnormalities (giving rise to the old term *Mongoloid*), mental retardation, shortened hands and trunk, and often defects in internal organs, including the heart. This problem is very rarely hidden in the mother's or father's own genetic makeup. Usually it is caused by incomplete chromosome separation in forming the individual egg or sperm from which the baby is formed. This incomplete separation leaves the egg with an extra, doubled-up chromosome, usually chromosome twenty-one. Problems with the sperm are uncommon (though some studies implicate paternal age as a factor). But the chance of having a doubling of chromosomes in the egg definitely increases with the mother's age.

A woman's body is born with all the eggs she will ever have. These eggs are not regenerated; rather, the original eggs mature over the mother's lifetime. Each month one or two eggs mature and are released for possible fertilization. As the mother grows older, the egg maturation process tends to go wrong slightly more often. Chromosome number twenty-one has a higher risk of being doubled. There is no age at which the risk of bearing a Down's syndrome child is zero. As a matter of fact, about half the children affected with this condition are born to mothers under thirty-five years old. This is because the birth rates are higher for younger women, though the chances of bearing an affected child are lower.

How much the incidence of birth defects caused by chromosomal abnormalities increases with age depends upon which study you read and who is being counted. Because it is not compulsory for physicians to report the occurrence of birth defects, national data generally reflect under-reporting. Despite the differences in reported statistics, approximate rates of risk by age are available for Down's syndrome. A thirty-year-old woman can expect a risk of 1 in 800; a thirty-five-year-old, 1 in 300; a forty-year-old, 1 in 100 live births.

Down's syndrome risks reported by the University of California at San Francisco Medical Center's genetic counselors are slightly higher, reflecting their experience with women at sixteen to eighteen weeks of pregnancy. Their estimates range from 1 in 100 at age thirty-five to 1 in 50 at age forty. In spite of higher risk at increasing age, chromosomal defects (most commonly Down's syndrome) can be diagnosed in utero. Thus, women who choose to become pregnant in later years can, through amniocentesis and chorionic villi sampling (described below) and subsequent selective abortion, substantially reduce this increased risk.

Another genetically linked risk related to age is the increased chance of fraternal twin births, caused by the release of two eggs at once. Most twin births are perfectly normal, but there are some potential medical risks associated with multiple births (low-birth-weight babies, for example). The incidence of twin births peaks at a maternal age of thirty-seven. A white woman of thirty-seven who has borne at least one other child has over twice the chance (16.8 cases of twinning in 1,000 birth events) of bearing twins than a woman of twenty has (6.3 cases of twinning in 1,000 birth events).

The incidence of stillbirths and miscarriages also rises with age. One study of 44,000 pregnancies shows the stillbirth and miscarriage rate for white women aged twenty to thirty to be 12 per 1,000. For thirty- to forty-year-olds the rate rose to 27 per 1,000. There were 49 miscarriages and stillbirths per 1,000 in the forty- to fifty-year-old range. The numbers for black women were similar but slightly higher, starting at 13 per 1,000 at twenty to thirty years old and going to 53 per 1,000 at forty to fifty.

Some of this increase may be due to general medical problems of the mother, but a large portion of it is probably genetic. There is some natural selection in pregnancies. For example, doctors believe that 21 percent to 24 percent of Down's syndrome fetuses are miscarried, and that as many as 50 percent of all conceptions end in spontaneous abortion (miscarriage).

Do older women have more problems with fetal development, in addition to facing these genetic risks? Probably not.

Some researchers feel that older women's placentas function poorly, giving rise to miscarriages. If this were true, then one would expect other types of birth defects to be common in children of older women. But only Down's syndrome, twinning, and miscarriage seem to be clearly age-related. Table 1 lists some problems of pregnancy and whether or not they are age-related.

Complications of Pregnancy and Their Relation to Age

**PREEXISTING DISORDERS
AGGRAVATED BY PREGNANCY**

Anemia	Not related to age.
Diabetes	Adverse effects cumulative over life-span.
Fibroid tumors	Incidence increases with age.
Hypertension/Cardio-vascular disease	Incidence increases with age.
Malnutrition	Not related to age.
Obesity	Not related to age.
Thyroid problems	Not related to age.

OBSTETRICAL COMPLICATIONS

During early pregnancy

Ectopic pregnancy	Not related to age.
Spontaneous abortion (miscarriage)	Incidence increases with age.

Pregnancy carried to term

Toxemia of pregnancy (preeclampsia and eclampsia)	Most common among teen-age mothers. Incidence related to high blood pressure, therefore indirectly to age; incidence also higher among first pregnancies.
Hemorrhage from placenta previa	Incidence increases with age and with parity.
Hemorrhage from placenta abruptio	Not related to age; incidence increases with parity.
Postpartum hemorrhage	Not directly related to age.
Sepsis (Infection)	Not related to age.

During labor and delivery

Dysfunctional labor	Incidence increases with age.
Prolonged labor	Not related to age.

Table 1

Risks to the Mother

What about the risk to the mother? Is it less safe for an older woman to give birth? The answer to that is a qualified yes. The older woman faces greater overall medical risk, because the incidence of most physical problems increases with age.

Medical literature divides complications of pregnancy and childbirth into two main categories: constitutional complications, which arise from the aggravation of preexisting disorders; and obstetrical complications, which arise only from the temporary condition of pregnancy.

Among the preexisting diseases that can complicate pregnancy, diabetes, fibroid tumors, and cardiovascular disease are of particular concern for women over thirty. The likelihood of these diseases increases with age, and the severity of diabetes also tends to increase with age. The risks of toxemia of pregnancy (a severe metabolic imbalance), postpartum hemorrhage, and postpartum infection increase for the older diabetic woman.

Some women are not diabetic until they get pregnant. There is a condition called gestational diabetes, in which a healthy, nondiabetic woman has diabetic symptoms when pregnant. She may even need insulin, though the need for the drug will disappear after delivery.

Forty percent of the women who have gestational diabetes will develop adult-onset diabetes within ten years of giving birth. It may be that the stresses of pregnancy simply accelerate (temporarily) a hereditary tendency to adult-onset diabetes. Every pregnant woman should have a urine test for diabetes. Luckily, adult-onset and gestational diabetes can often be handled without insulin, by changes in diet.

Fibroids are benign uterine tumors that occur with more frequency as women age. They usually have no effect on pregnancy, though occasionally they may grow large enough to endanger the fetus, causing miscarriage or difficulties at delivery. Since fibroids cause little problem to the nonpregnant woman, she may not know she has them unless she gets a prepregnancy pelvic examination and specifically asks her doctor about their presence. Also, hypertension (high blood pressure) and cardiovascular conditions are serious diseases that become more common with age.

Any woman who has diabetes, problems with fibroids, hypertension, heart disease, anemia, or obesity should confer with a physician before becoming pregnant. Her health status should be assessed, and if she does get pregnant, she should choose a concerned obstetrician who will carefully monitor her pregnancy. As with all other risks, good health care can reduce the likelihood that these conditions will cause complications during pregnancy.

Many constitutional complications, as above, increase with age. Most obstetrical complications do not increase. Toxemia (often related to obesity, hypertension, or diabetes) does tend to increase somewhat with age, but it is also common among teen-age mothers. Other conditions, such as ectopic pregnancy, a pregnancy in which the fertilized egg implants outside the uterus, are very dangerous, but the incidence of these conditions does not increase with age.

The end of pregnancy is labor. Statistics seem to support the assumption that older first-time mothers have more problems than younger women with dysfunctional labor—that is, labor that does not seem to "work" effectively toward birth. But there is some evidence that this higher rate of labor complications may be due, at least in part, to the fact that the older mother can expect more conservative treatment in the labor and delivery room. While there is no significant difference in length of labor between older and younger mothers, older mothers tend to have more cesareans. In one study, women over thirty-five were five times more likely to be delivered by cesarean section, even though in two out of three cases the indications for cesarean delivery were questionable.

Because of this cautious medical response to the potentially "high risk" over-thirty-five first-time mothers, women should carefully discuss labor and delivery expectations with their physicians. Doctors have a heavy responsibility to do the absolute best thing for the mother and baby, a responsibility enforced by the malpractice courts. A doctor may use preventative medical procedures, such as cesarean delivery, that have not been anticipated by a woman who has prepared for a natural birth. Disappointment with the birth experience may result. It is therefore best to have an honest understanding with the obstetrician and a realistic view of modern medical practice and its constraints.

HOW TO REDUCE THE RISKS FOR MOTHER AND BABY

To have a healthy child, it is best to be a healthy woman. Before conceiving, a woman of any age should assess her general health and current habits. Pay special attention to the following areas of potential concern:

- weight
- exercise level
- diet
- use of drugs (including alcohol and smoking)
- chronic or medical problems (such as high blood pressure or herpes infection)
- exposure to environmental dangers (chemicals, viruses)
- family history of both mother- and father-to-be.

Many over-thirty women choose to have a health evaluation by their gynecologist or family doctor before attempting to become pregnant. Women of any age who have a chronic disease such as diabetes, heart disease, high blood pressure, genital herpes, or cancer in a state of cure or remission, *should* consult with a doctor before attempting pregnancy. For most older women, though, the pre-pregnancy consultation is more optional than necessary. The doctor can check that nothing obvious is wrong, take a medical history, and advise on diet and lifestyle. If something worrisome or suspicious is found, it may well be possible to cure the condition before you get pregnant.

Weight: You should be close to your ideal weight before becoming pregnant. This does not mean that you *must* lose that five pounds or get back to a size-ten dress before daring pregnancy. Five to twenty pounds above the "perfect" weight is not an issue here. On the other hand, serious maternal obesity definitely increases the risk of complications.

Exercise level: Reasonable exercise is healthy. But marathon running and other sports that require intense training can cause disruptions in the ovulation cycle and make pregnancy more difficult to achieve.

Diet: They used to say, "Lose a tooth for every baby." People don't say that anymore, since most women are careful about what they eat while pregnant, and they try to get enough calcium for themselves and the baby. But don't wait until you are pregnant to begin to eat right. Give up strenuous dieting and also give up junk food, *before* you become pregnant. Be in good nutritional shape early, ready for the first few months of pregnancy when your appetite may be depressed. Also, many women are slightly iron-deficient, a condition that can easily be corrected before pregnancy. Your doctor can advise you on proper diet as well as weight gain while you are pregnant.

Use of drugs: Concerning prescription drugs, your doctor is your best guide as to what you should take and what you might want to do without. Regarding over-the-counter drugs, avoid as many as possible and talk to your doctor about any you wish to continue taking while pregnant. You may be advised to stop taking them or to substitute related drugs that are not dangerous to the fetus. If you are taking birth control pills, discontinue them a few months before attempting to conceive, and use a condom or diaphragm for the intervening months. This will allow your body to restore its own hormonal balance before pregnancy begins.

Then there are the recreational drugs: nicotine, alcohol, caffeine, street drugs. Smoking and alcohol are both associated with a higher rate of birth defects. Smokers' babies tend to have low birth weights. The statistics show a virtual doubling of risk that the baby will weigh under five pounds if the mother smokes. In a sample of 1,000 mothers who do not smoke, 51 low-birth-weight babies can be expected; for mothers who do smoke, the rate is 92.4 per 1,000.

Maternal smoking continues to be linked to sickness and death for children throughout early childhood. A recent literature review on smoking and pregnancy showed that the death rate for children between one month and five years was 3.9 per 1,000 for maternal nonsmokers, and more than twice that—9.6 per 1,000—for maternal smokers. It is not clear whether this higher death rate is due to a higher rate of congenital malformations, or to more severe upper-respiratory-tract infections (a well-known health hazard for smokers' children), or to other causes. Nevertheless, the trend is consistent throughout pregnancy, birth, and early childhood. *Give up smoking.* It is the best thing you can do for your baby.

Alcohol use, at the rate of several drinks a day, also has an adverse effect on the fetus. Fetal alcohol syndrome (FAS) is a birth defect that leads to characteristic facial features (small head, flattened features, upturned nose, wide-spread eyes), and mental and physical retardation. According to a recent estimate, one child out of 750 is born with fetal alcohol syndrome. FAS is one of the leading causes of mental retardation in the United States. Unlike Down's syndrome, however, it is completely preventable, simply by not drinking during pregnancy. Even small amounts of alcohol are believed to have bad effects on the developing fetus.

A word about caffeine: Early studies showed that caffeine could affect fetal development. Later studies attacked the early studies, pointing out that the earlier studies did not take the smoking and drinking habits of the women into account. Women who drink a lot of coffee are also more likely to smoke and drink alcohol. To really assess the effects of caffeine, it would be necessary to hold other variables constant.

At this time, it doesn't seem that caffeine is particularly hazardous. It is unlikely that it is more hazardous than some herb teas, for example, with their combinations of relatively untested ingredients. When in doubt, use moderation in all things.

The effects of illegal street drugs are also difficult to quantify. Some research shows that marijuana cigarettes, like tobacco cigarettes, are associated with low-birth-weight babies. Other drugs are also dangerous. Babies of heroin addicts can be born addicted to heroin (and many are born that way every day in this country). This certainly implies that street drugs, like other drugs, can cross the placental barrier and affect fetal development.

Be sure your doctor is fully informed of the drugs you are taking, both at the prepregnancy checkup and throughout your pregnancy. This way, you will be offered the information necessary to help you protect your baby from damaging substances.

Chronic or medical problems: These must be discussed with your doctor. Most women who have heart disease, hypertension, or diabetes are aware of these conditions if they have had regular medical checkups. If you are not in the habit of regular checkups, definitely get one before attempting to get pregnant. These conditions make pregnancy truly high-risk, and careful medical supervision of the pregnancy becomes absolutely essential.

A chronic problem extremely dangerous for the baby deserves special mention here: genital herpes. Women who have genital herpes sometimes pass it to their babies at the moment of birth. It is an absolutely devastating infection for a newborn infant, resulting in death within a few days of birth in about 50 percent of the cases. If a woman has, or has ever had genital herpes, she should inform her doctor of the problem; she may also consider cesarean delivery to avoid infecting the baby, if there is active infection at the time of delivery.

Exposure to environmental dangers: This is a difficult subject, because our modern world is so full of chemicals, many of which are dangerous to the developing fetus. If you work in a hazardous chemical or radiation area, it is best to transfer out of the area while pregnant. The dangerous area doesn't have to be a chemical plant: anesthesiologists and beauticians may also be at risk. Remember, too, that many lawn and garden chemicals (weed killers and insecticides) contain hazardous compounds. When in doubt ask your doctor, or allow someone else to handle the chemicals.

Exposure to viruses is more difficult to control. Lots of people have colds and flus, and catching them is one of the hazards of living. Try to avoid associating with sick people while pregnant; you and your baby do deserve some special consideration at this time. Also avoid cat droppings, bird droppings, and eating raw meat while pregnant. These materials can carry toxoplasmosis, a disease dangerous to the fetus. While pregnant, have someone else clean the litter box and the bird cage, and avoid steak tartare.

Family history: Is there diabetes in your family or in the family of the baby's father? Is your family from eastern Europe, and are you Jewish (one in twenty-five Jews from eastern Europe is a carrier for Tay-Sachs disease)? Does someone in your family have thalassemia? These are all genetically inherited diseases, and your doctor may well advise you to see a genetic counselor. If you are over thirty-five, and therefore at higher risk for carrying a Down's syndrome baby, you may also be encouraged to see a counselor.

Genetic counseling is a very new profession. Only recently has it been possible to check healthy people for the presence of dangerous genes (usually through blood tests). Not all common genetic diseases can be detected this way, but research continues to progress in this area. More complete genetic reviews will undoubtedly be possible in the future.

Discussion of the parents' genetic history is only one step in genetic counseling. The second step occurs after pregnancy: reviewing the genetic makeup of the unborn child. This review is usually undertaken through amniocentesis, and it is excellent at detecting Down's syndrome, the major age-related genetic concern of older mothers, as well as determining the presence or absence of other genetic disorders.

Amniocentesis and the Older Mother

For amniocentesis, the doctor takes a sample of the amniotic fluid surrounding the fetus. The sample is withdrawn by a needle carefully inserted through the mother's abdomen into the uterus. First the doctor determines the position of the fetus by ultrasound, so that the needle can avoid any contact with the fetus. The length of the needle may be daunting, but the procedure is rarely painful. While many women do have cramps afterward, the procedure poses no known danger for the woman and very little for the fetus.

Some say that amniocentesis increases the rate of miscarriage. But any effect it has on this rate is very small— so small that as many studies indicate it has no effect as indicate it has a slight effect. For example, in one study of 1,000 women who had amniocentesis and 990 who did not have it, the spontaneous abortion rate was 3.2 percent for those who did not have the procedure and 3.5 percent for those who did. This degree of variation is not statistically significant. Another study showed a "less than 1 percent" rate of problems. When there is a very low incidence rate, it is hard to really assess the risk, except to say that it is small. Many doctors believe that the amount of risk is directly associated with the skill of the practitioner. It is wise to have the procedure performed in a large medical center, by a specialist.

After the doctor removes about one fluid ounce of amniotic fluid, it is sent to the lab to be analyzed. The fluid consists of a mixture of amnionical water and a few skin cells that the fetus has sloughed off. The few fetal cells are separated from the water in a centrifuge, and then they are grown in a cell culture medium until there is enough material to analyze. This cell culturing takes three to four weeks. The results yield information on chromosomal abnormalities, and they also reveal the sex of the infant.

For most women, waiting for the results of the culture is the most stressful time of the pregnancy. The test is usually performed sometime between the sixteenth and eighteenth week after the last menstrual period, but the results aren't ready till two to four weeks later. By then, the movements of the baby in the womb are readily apparent to the mother, and yet the decision on abortion remains in the future. It is all worth it, however, for the 98 to 99 percent of women who are told that the defects in question are not present. They can truly relax, confident of carrying a baby without Down's syndrome and enjoy the rest of their pregnancy.

The 1 to 2 percent who must face bad news generally accept that it was a matter of hearing it now or hearing it later. They would have discovered the problem at the birth of the child, at which time it would have been no easier— and sometimes harder—to take. This is not to imply that their decision on abortion, whether they choose it or not, is an easy one. Some physicians feel that no woman should have amniocentesis unless she has considered and accepted the possibility of abortion. Others suggest that even if abortion is out of the question, the foreknowledge of any problem can be helpful. Of course, considering abortion in late pregnancy is quite different from considering it dispassionately while not pregnant. The fact remains that carrying a handicapped child is always an unhappy situation, no matter when or in what circumstances the parents find out.

What is needed is a way of finding out earlier, so that more of the pregnancy can be relaxing and nobody has to face a second-trimester abortion. A method for doing this is under development and is now available in many medical centers: chorionic villi sampling. Samples are taken of the villi (small projections) into the lining of the uterus, which are the basis for the placental attachment. The procedure is performed seven weeks after the last menstrual period. Because the villi are part of the developing placenta and because they started from the same cell as the fetus, no cell culturing is required. The sample, as taken, is sufficient for chromosomal analysis, and results are often available within forty-eight hours.

Chorionic villi sampling seems to present very little risk to the mother and is virtually painless. It can be performed in a doctor's office and requires no anesthetic. The sample is taken with a small vaginal catheter. Nevertheless, chorionic villae sampling (CVS) seems to cause slightly more miscarriages than amniocentesis does. Preliminary estimates are that CVS triggers a miscarriage at a rate of 1 to 3 percent, while amniocentesis triggers miscarriage at a rate of below 1 percent. CVS also cannot detect some conditions (spina bifida, for example) that amniocentesis can, although these conditions can be diagnosed in a blood test of the mother later in pregnancy (the alpha-fetoprotein test).

It would be nice if *everything* could be detected so simply; giving a little blood is easy on the mother and certainly has no effect on the miscarriage rate. Research microbiologists at Michigan State University are trying to develop a blood test that could substitute for both amniocentesis and CVS. So far, their research results have been very encouraging, but it is not clear whether they will continue to have success (they have tested only two women) and whether their method can be adapted from the research laboratory to an everyday, repeatable procedure.

The Well-Informed Mother-to-Be

Overall, a well-informed, healthy woman who takes an active role in ensuring her health during preconception and pregnancy and who has high-quality medical care has excellent chances of a safe and normal pregnancy and delivery. The secret of a healthy pregnancy is knowledge, good medical care, and the willingness to do what is necessary to provide the best conditions for nurturing a healthy baby. Involvement and willingness are not age-dependent, and the outcome is rarely age-dependent.

Can We Afford a Baby?

Nobody can afford a baby. It doesn't matter how much money you make, you still can't afford one: Having more money simply means spending more money.

Babies are no good as tax shelters, either. The deduction of $1,000 will net only $500 in tax savings, even in a high tax bracket. It would be much better to buy a new house or set up an IRA or a Keogh. No investment counselor will ever suggest a strategic move into parenthood.

And if you want simple adoration with minimum cash investment, dogs are available for free at your local animal shelter. Vet bills are lower than doctor bills, and no day-care expenses are incurred.

Nobody has a baby for any rational reason. People have a baby because they want a baby. Their reasons are emotional, sentimental, deep. That is why Chapter 6, on making the decision, attempts to help people get in touch with their most profound hopes and emotions. There are no calculations of interest rates in that chapter.

After having been "rational" for thirty years, it is hard to start making decisions in another mode. So often, it has been appropriate to plan, to think ahead: "This job will lead to an opportunity for the kind of job I want." Or "I have to save $200 a month in order to take that trip to the West Coast this spring." These are all rational statements. They show managerial competence and planning ability. They have very little to do with choosing to have a baby.

Nobody can plan for the expenses of raising a child, because nobody can predict what those expenses will be. Will the child be a boy or a girl? Will it be healthy or have a physical problem that needs attention? Will the mother wish she could stay home more, or will she be eager to get back to the world of work? There are some things you just can't know until they happen, and almost everything involved with babies falls into that category.

To get some perspective on current-day planning for a baby, it is worthwhile looking at how children were raised in the past. Panic at the financial aspect of parenthood is perfectly reasonable. The economic burden of child-rearing has never been as great as it is now.

RURAL AND URBAN CHILDREN: ECONOMICS VERSUS EMOTIONS

Throughout most of the rural world, children, especially boys, are considered an economic asset. It is an economic tragedy for a farm couple to be childless.

For rural people, having children is a decision of both the head and the heart. (The term *decision* is used advisedly. When birth control is introduced to a third-world area, family size usually doesn't change much; people still want large families.)

Is this way of looking at children part of the agrarian past or a specialty of less-developed nations? William doesn't think so. He grew up on a dairy farm in Oregon in the 1970s, and he was an economic asset to his family, whether he wanted to be or not. He still vividly remembers being forced to quit the high school wrestling team ("The only sport I ever did well in; I've always been small and skinny, but in my weight class I was really good!") in order to be home in time to do chores.

Most suburban parents would have been absolutely delighted to see their undersized son enjoying a sport. They would have let nothing interfere with this part of his development. But William's dad was concerned with keeping the farm, not with the possibility of needing to provide expensive child psychologists if his son didn't adjust. This is a common rural view of the value of children.

Though this view of children hurt William in high school, other parts of his rural upbringing also helped turn him into a very successful young engineer. He was an economic asset to his family rather than a financial drain, and knowing he was needed on the farm increased his self-esteem.

Of course, not all children live in the country, and most urban children are not economic assets to their families. But during the baby boom they weren't such incredible economic liabilities, either.

The parents of the baby boom grew up during the Depression, then lived through World War II. When these outside forces on their lives finally subsided, both men and women really wanted a home and children.

New families formed, and there was no place for them to go. Many a new baby was brought home to a "temporary housing" Quonset hut or an overcrowded apartment or the grandparents' house. The fathers and mothers who raised the baby-boom generation did not always have an easy time. But in some ways having children was easier, if only because the parents' expectations were not so high.

Even a small two-bedroom apartment seemed luxurious in 1950, after the three years a young mother might have spent with her parents while her husband was in the service. Many families did not even own a car; as late as 1960, a quarter of American families were carless. Two cars in a family were a luxury of the rich. There was no shame attached to living in a small apartment, parking the stroller in the middle of the living room, having the baby and two toddlers sleep in the second bedroom. That's how almost everybody was living. Middle-class people were content to raise children in conditions that might be considered a mark of poverty today. And if the family did own a house, the mortgage payment calculation would not have been predicated on the wife's income, as we mentioned in the first chapter.

Some of the gains in living standards since those days are real, but some have been illusory. Over half the families in the country today may have two cars, but over half the mothers also work, and need that second car to commute. A well-equipped, modern kitchen, with microwave and dishwasher, definitely saves time for the cook. On the other hand, it doesn't save forty hours a week for the working mother.

People may have been poorer, but they also gave up less in order to have children during the baby boom. Today, people are richer, and there is more to give up. Or perhaps there just seems to be more to lose.

IRRELEVANT STATISTICS—AND SOME RELEVANT LIFESTYLES

The easiest way to convince yourself that nobody can afford a baby is to look at the statistics. Those published in 1982 suggest that it will cost anywhere from $30,000 to $250,000 to raise a child. The lower numbers are for rural children, the higher numbers for children of affluent, urban families.

What can be done about these outrageous figures? It is clear that financial planning for the child's entire life is impractical. You can no more "save up" for raising a child than you can save the entire price of a house before purchasing it.

And for another thing, these estimates are misleading. Having a baby forces certain changes in the adults' lifestyles, some caused by the economic consequences of having a child, some by the emotional consequences. For example, people with a child have more incentive to buy a house, save for college, take "family-style" vacations. Are these financial consequences or changes in priorities? If one assumes that parents want to do the same things with their money that nonparents want to do, the "costs" of a child are extremely high. If one assumes that the parents' own priorities will be changed by the experience of caring for another human being, then you notice that babies don't eat much, and it is what you *want* to provide for your children that makes the difference.

Families' spending habits are as varied as the families themselves. Some buy their clothes at Saks, others at thrift stores. Some mothers work only part-time at lucrative jobs, giving up tens of thousands of dollars a year in possible full-time earnings. Other mothers never intended to work at all and do not consider loss of earnings part of the cost of children.

Instead of looking at such statistics, it is better to look at how real families spend their money. In a brief survey by the *San Francisco Chronicle* in 1982, a high-income family estimated that they spent $29,000 a year raising their two boys (ages eleven and eight). The income of this family was not stated in the article, but was probably around $70,000 per year. The child-care expenses included $6,-300 for private-school tuition, $700 for clothing, $3,600 for food at home, and $3,400 a year for entertainment. (The entertainment expense includes the children's share in a summer home.) To a certain extent, the private school is a child-care expense, since it provides extended after-school day care for the youngsters, allowing their mother to work.

In the same article, a family with an annual income of $19,000 estimates that they spend $7,500 a year on their two girls, a five-year-old and a nine-month-old. This includes $1,200 for food at home, $360 for clothing, $2,400 on child care so the mother can work part-time, nothing on education, and $240 on entertainment (an occasional movie, books, crayons). While the total is not high compared with $29,000, it is huge compared with the family's resources.

Both the families spent a little less than half their income on their children. This does not mean, however, that if they didn't have children, there would be twice as much money for the adults. While there would definitely be more money, it is unlikely that things would divide so simply; somehow, instead of the money covering four people in the family, it would cover two people. Without the children there would be such different spending habits entirely that comparisons would often prove misleading.

But down to the nitty-gritty of the actual expenses: In the stated costs, child care is one of the largest. Before a child is born, a woman's income is a simple plus for the family. After the child is born, there are trade-offs. If the mother's job was low-paying to begin with, it may not be economical for her to continue to work. As a rule of thumb, the mother should earn two-and-a-half to three times the cost of quality child care. If she does not earn that much, it may make economic sense for her to stay home. Besides the obvious costs of taxes, work clothes, and commuting are the hidden costs of fatigue: hurried shopping and convenience-food meals. Fatigue can cost a surprising amount.

Of course, many mothers prefer to work, even if they are not netting very much money. But women who are working "for the satisfaction of it" rather than for the money usually prefer to work part-time. A forty-hour-a-week job at the office plus another one at home is just too stressful, unless there is extra money to alleviate some of the problems.

Reasonable financial planning for a baby does not mean saving up for the entire "extra" costs of a family-oriented life. This is something that evolves, not something you plan for. Nonetheless, some advance planning can be extremely useful, especially when it concerns making the first few months after the child is born easier, at least financially. You need time to adjust to the baby without worrying about money at the same time.

DOLLARS AND INFANTS

The purpose of financial planning is to allow the family some flexibility after the baby is born. There are few things in the world more wrenching than *having* to go back to work within four weeks, whether you want to or not, in order to avoid foreclosure on your house. It can also be aggravating to realize that you could have gotten more disability payments, if only you had handled the application process correctly. It would be devastating to find out that your individual health insurance policy doesn't cover the baby's medical expenses, especially if the baby has a health problem.

There are four types of planning to concern yourself with before the baby is born. Although the four progressive steps are interrelated, they are different enough to be discussed separately.

The first two steps are planning for the delivery in the hospital and for the baby's arrival at home. This includes making sure your health insurance will cover the newborn and knowing what portion of the hospital and doctor bills you will have to pay out of your own pocket. It also includes being ready to take the baby home: having a crib or cradle, diapers, a few changes of clothes for the baby, nursing bras if you are nursing, bottles if you are bottle feeding, and so on.

The third and fourth steps involve planning for your minimum leave and possibly your extended leave from work. What disability payments are you entitled to, those first few weeks after the baby is born? What is the company's policy on maternity leave? How much money can you expect to have coming into the house for those first few weeks? Can you manage on that? And how long can you reasonably stay at home with your baby before returning to work?

All these questions should be answered earlier rather than later. A little forethought can save a lot of aggravation.

The Hospital Stay

Simply listing the medical and hospital costs of a birth is frightening, but it is usually irrelevent. The question is not how much it costs, but rather how much you will have to pay personally and how much your insurance will cover. Worrying about the overall rise in health-care costs can be left to the newspaper columnists, who get paid to interpret such things. In the meantime, it will pay you to understand your health insurance benefits and how they relate to your probable expenses.

First, review your health insurance policy. Does it have maternity benefits? Does it cover the baby? What costs does it pay, and what doesn't it pay? Some of the things you should consider:

- the preexisting conditions clause
- whether it is a family policy plan
- coinsured payments
- benefits coverage

The Preexisting Conditions Clause

If you move or change jobs during your pregnancy or if your company changes insurance carriers, you may be caught by the "preexisting conditions" clause. Most insurers will not cover conditions that existed before the policy took effect. There may be a waiting period, after which preexisting conditions will be covered when a year has elapsed from the first date the policy went into effect. This clause protects insurance companies from people who would buy a policy as soon as they find out they have an expensive disease. It also protects the companies against paying for many labors and deliveries. Insurance companies can be somewhat arbitrary on how they use their preexisting conditions clause. If you plan to get pregnant within the first year of coverage, we advise that you check the policy of your carrier.

The preexisting conditions clause makes it impossible to get a better insurance policy while pregnant. If, after you become pregnant, you find that your current policy leaves several important expenses uncovered by insurance, you will have to use your savings to pay for those items yourself.

Therefore, you want to enter pregnancy with a stable insurance history and keep the same carriers throughout the pregnancy and birth period. It is usually unwise to change jobs or to move from state to state while pregnant. This is especially important for the single woman or the woman whose husband may not be working full-time. Your husband should also probably keep the same job over the course of your pregnancy. Otherwise, you may lose more in health benefits than you could possibly gain by not waiting the several necessary months to make the job or geographical change.

A company that changes insurance carriers will usually protect its workers (such as yourself, who might get pregnant during this time) by insisting that the "preexisting conditions" clause be stricken from the new carrier's contract. Nevertheless, one woman whose company changed insurance plans put it this way: "The new insurance company *eventually* paid me for the hospital bill. But they turned down my first two applications, claiming the pregnancy was a 'preexisting condition.' I had to have the personnel department help me deal with those guys. And of course, I'm getting the dunning letters from the hospital, while the insurers keep getting interest on the money they should have paid. Frankly, I think it's a bit of a racket."

Family-Policy Plan

An individual health plan, covering only the individual, should be converted to a family policy (usually at your expense) before the baby is born. Many women are covered by individual health insurance, with the premium paid by their employer. Such a policy usually doesn't pay for a child's health care or hospital expense. *This coverage is essential.* If the baby has any health problem, the costs can be astronomical. Expenses of over $1,000 a day in an intensive care nursery are not uncommon.

Coinsured Payments

Many policies have "coinsured" payments. That is, the insurer will pay 80 percent of the cost and the "coinsurer" will pay the other 20 percent. When there is only one policy in a family, the family itself is the coinsurer, paying 20 percent of the costs, as well as an almost certain "deductible" fee (deductible for the insurance company, that is, as in "all expenses over $200 are split 80–20 with the coinsurer"). If both husband and wife work, and if they both have separate comprehensive health policies, the husband's insurance company may pay the "coinsured" part of the expenses, and perhaps the deductible. Of course, there may be some costs that neither policy pays (see benefits coverage, below). With two policies, however, one paying 80 percent of the bill and the other paying the 20 percent "coinsured" part of the bill, your chances of having almost 100 percent coverage of your medical expenses is increased.

Benefits Coverage

Most policies have a scale of how much medical services are supposed to cost and will cover 80 percent of that amount. If you live in a high-cost urban area, birth and delivery may cost more than they allow. You will then have to pay 20 percent of the costs they allow, as well as all of the difference between the costs they allow and reality. How much will that be? For example, you might find that your doctor charges $1,600 for a cesarean and that the medical insurance uses $1,400 as its "reasonable and customary fee." In this case, the insurance would pay 80 percent of $1,400, or $1,120, and you would pay the difference of $480 ($280 for your 20 percent coinsurance, plus $200 that the doctor charged you but the insurance company did not cover, because it was above the "reasonable and customary" fee).

If you choose to have nontraditional medical care (for example, birth in your home) these costs are rarely covered by your medical insurance.

Most policies will not pay for genetic counseling, private hospital rooms, newborn exam by pediatrician, or circumcision. Some will not pay for newborn well-baby hospital care.

You should determine, through your doctor and hospital, the typical charges for an uncomplicated labor and delivery, as well as for a cesarean. Then determine, either with the help of your personnel department or directly from the insurance carrier, how much will be covered. It takes time and effort to do this, but persevere! You do have some control, after all, on how you want your baby born. You can choose your doctor and your hospital. They should cooperate with you on determining costs. The business of delivering babies has never been more market oriented (perhaps because there are so many mature women who insist on knowing the facts). In some areas, hospitals are wooing prospective maternity patients with gifts, special-price packages, and candlelight steak-and-champagne dinners.

Many hospitals will give you all sorts of useful financial information in a preregistration packet. (They may also insist on a preregistration fee, usually $500 due two months before your delivery date.) When you get a preregistration packet, study it carefully. Bring it to your personnel department for help in understanding what is covered.

Not understanding the hospital costs can lead to much anxiety in the first few months. Hospitals frequently deal with people who are in financial straits due to illness, and the hospitals have money problems of their own. Therefore, even when mercy is part of the hospital's name, the administrators are likely to be very unsympathetic about people not meeting their payments. If your bill is being paid through federal programs, the hospital may wait for payment. If you are middle class, however, and you've simply misunderstood your insurance coverage, the hospital is unlikely to be thoughtful of either your nerves or your other money problems. Plan ahead, and avoid the stress that comes with large, unpaid hospital bills.

Some typical medical care costs, as of this writing, follow:

Major Costs

- Doctor, prenatal care and normal delivery $1,000
- Doctor, prenatal care and cesarean delivery $1,500–$2,000
- Hospital stay, mother, two days $1,500 to $4,000
- Hospital stay, well baby, two days (many insurance policies will not cover this) $500
- Hospital for mother, five days, cesarean $5,500
- Hospital for baby, five days, cesarean $1,250
- Alternative Birth Center (in hospital) normal delivery and twelve-hour stay for mother and baby after delivery $1,000

Minor or Hidden Costs
(that insurance won't usually pay)

- Husband's meals while he is visiting
- The cost of a TV in the room
- Telephone use (often with a surcharge)
- Private or semiprivate room, if insurance covers only a ward (even if a ward isn't available)
- Extra time in recovery room (depending on circumstances)
- Staying even a few minutes beyond discharge time (may add up to a full day's hospitalization, which the insurance will probably not pay)

Some insurance companies are now giving mothers a $100 cash rebate if they check out of the hospital within twelve hours of the birth.

Overall, planning ahead will probably save you money, especially if your planning involves arranging for adequate insurance. It will certainly save you the grief and aggravation of unexpected expenses in the first few months you are home. Which brings us to the second step: planning to bring baby home.

Bringing Baby Home

In order to bring baby home from the hospital, you will need

- a place for the baby to sleep (with bedding)
- travel equipment (car seat, baby carrier)
- clothes and receiving blankets
- feeding equipment
- diapers.

Luckily, there are only two major expenditures in this list: a good crib and a good car seat. Various ways to cut costs can be easily found for many of the other things on the list.

Making Room

Preparing a place for baby at home is cheap compared with the hospital bill. But of course it *can* be *made* expensive. Saks Fifth Avenue offers upscale layette clothes and baby equipment, and elsewhere, designer cribs and $200 strollers are common. Keep in mind, that fancy things are for parents' pride, not baby's happiness. Let grandparents and friends take care of the extravagant little goodies. For yourself, concentrate on the basics.

You may not be able to set aside a separate room for your baby, but the space you do have should be bright and cheerful. The area may have secondhand furniture for you (a rocking chair is very useful), but do get a good-quality crib for the baby. Since 1974, when the U.S. Consumer Product Safety Commission set special standards, cribs have been made with slats that are no more than 2 ⅜ inches apart, to prevent neck entrapment. Don't buy or borrow a used crib unless you know that you are getting a good, recent model that has no slats missing and is designed to meet the 1974 federal guidelines.

The crib mattress should be fairly firm and fit snugly into the crib so that the baby cannot wedge his head between the slats and the mattress. Babies don't need pillows. But they do need several changes of bedding: mattress protectors, mattress pads, fitted crib sheets, and blankets.

Babies tend to accumulate so much "stuff" that they need their own chest of drawers. Some people also like to have a changing table; others always change the baby in her crib or on the counter in the bathroom.

It is often convenient if the new baby can sleep in the parents' bedroom for a few weeks. That is when cradles come into use. A better buy, however, might be a small traveling crib, which can be used in the bedroom for those first few weeks and then used when you are out visiting with the baby. Which brings us to traveling equipment.

The Traveling Baby

Two things are essential for a traveling baby. The first is a car seat. And we do mean the *first,* because many hospitals will not let you take the baby from the building unless they see that you have one. Some car seats convert for an older child; others are for an infant only. We have seen many a baby snooze happily in the infant-only type, which doubles as a carry-and-nap seat (and often adjusts from sitting-up to lying-down positions), and we tend to like those seats. The main purpose of the car seat is to keep the infant safe in the car, and both types (infant and convertible) that meet the 1981 federal regulations will do this. That is, they will keep the baby safe if they are properly installed. But remember, not all car seats fit well into all cars, so take your own car along and make sure the seat works before buying it.

The second thing you need is a way to carry the infant around the house or to the store without holding him in your hands all the time. For this, a front-pack for a little baby and a back-pack later are really useful (some brands will do both).

Strollers can come later. You don't need a stroller for the first few months, and you probably should only plan on buying it when the baby outgrows her front-pouch baby carrier.

Baby Clothes

Babies don't care what they are wearing, as long as they are dry and warm. Shopping at garage sales for baby clothes is a very good idea. It's nice if you know some mothers (from prenatal exercise class or Lamaze class) with slightly older babies. You can usually buy hand-me-downs from them.

Babies outgrow their clothes very rapidly. The reason that the stores carry newborn, 3-month, 6-month, 9-month, and 12-month sizes is that each set of clothes is good for three months or less. The layette clothes are hardly the only baby clothes you will have to purchase the first year, so don't spend much money on them. Also, avoid the prepackaged, prepriced "layette" set. It is sure to contain things you won't choose to use, duplicates of things you will get as gifts, and not enough of other clothes you wish you had.

Remember, too, that you are likely to get lots of newborn-size articles as gifts and shower presents. Don't overbuy. The world must be full of underused, outgrown newborn-sized outfits. By the time the baby is a few months old, you will know your own style of dressing the baby and be a more informed shopper in the 6-month size range.

Part of being an informed shopper is realizing that many children's "night" clothes (especially the cotton ones) are treated with fire-retardant chemicals. One of these chemicals (TRIS) was taken off the market in the late '70s, since it was suspected of causing cancer. The chemicals used now are probably safer. Some mothers, however, prefer to always dress their infants in untreated daytime-type clothes, to avoid contact with the treatment chemicals. Read the labels. If the piece of clothing has washing instructions designed to retain flame-retardant properties, it has been chemically treated. We are in favor of naturally flame-retardant materials for babies, rather than chemically treated materials. Table 2 lists recommended "starter" baby clothes.

Baby Clothes

- Four or five stretch suits.
- Sweater or jacket.
- Other clothes (nighties, booties, hats). Since most babies these days spend so much of their time in stretchies, go easy on the other clothes.
- Warm outer bunting or sleeping bag, if the weather is likely to be cold.
- Bedding: cribsheets, a waterproof crib mattress protector, two crib blankets, a few receiving blankets, and some flannelized rubber pads (these are for changing the baby, to put under the sheet in the crib or bassinet, and for putting on your lap when you are holding the baby).
- At least one baby bath towel with a hood (practical for swaddling a crying baby after her bath).

Table 2

Feeding Equipment

At first, babies only drink. You will eventually need a high chair, but you might as well wait until the baby sits up before buying it. (If you are cramped for space, portable baby seats are available that will fit right onto your table.) If you choose to breastfeed, you will need some nursing bras, some comfortable outfits (anything that buttons down the front is convenient, as are slacks and pull-over tops—just lift the top and tuck the baby under), and some vitamin supplements. Some mothers find a manual breast-pump very useful, along with a few bottles for relief feedings. Others find the pumps lead to sore and cracked nipples. If you are bottle feeding, you will need bottles, nipples, formula, and sterilizing equipment.

Diapers

Everybody needs both kinds of diapers. If you choose disposable diapers, you will still need a dozen of the cloth variety as burp cloths, to put on your shoulder when burping the baby. If you choose to use cloth diapers, you may still find the disposable ones easier and more convenient for the first hectic days at home, and absolutely necessary for taking the baby on outings. Overall, disposable diapers are more expensive than cloth but tend to be more convenient.

Toys

Don't buy a newborn many toys. More than 150,000 toys are now on the market, but an infant's abilities are too limited for him to appreciate much more than a crib mobile at first. Later, choose toys that are appropriate to your baby's age and skills and are simple, safe, and durable. Remember, too, that babies often actually prefer objects they find around the house. Many a mother has happily bought her crawling child a $20 toy only to find that her darling greatly preferred the box it came in. Don't let advertising fool you, either: No toy out there will automatically raise the IQ of your child.

Overall, there is no particular secret to shopping for a baby. Babies have special needs, such as cribs, but they don't need elaborate clothing or high-tech toys. You will probably want to buy your car seat and crib new, or else borrow them from people who bought them recently, in order to be sure they meet the most recent federal regulations. For everything else, garage sales and other mothers are probably your best and most economical sources. It is the care you put into the baby, not the money you spend on him, that counts.

Of course, to care for a new baby, you have to be home with him, at least for a couple of weeks. Which brings us to our third planning area.

Planning for Your Minimum Leave

It takes several weeks for the mother's body to readjust after childbirth. At the end of pregnancy, the uterus is one of the heaviest organs in the body, weighing almost three pounds. Then the uterus shrinks, giving rise to contractions called afterpains. Every contraction shrinks it further, and within six weeks the uterus weighs only about three ounces. These afterpains are less painful than labor but much more unpredictable. Recovery hurts.

Kidney function has also adjusted to pregnancy (excreting for two), but four weeks after birth it is back to normal. The genital region undergoes many changes: stitches heal, the labia become less swollen. Intercourse can usually resume four to six weeks after you have delivered. Hormonal levels also go through rapid change, as the pregnancy hormones are replaced by those of lactation (if the mother is nursing) or the usual monthly cycle (if she is not).

What does all this have to do with financial planning? These physical readjustments are the reason that a new mother needs six weeks' disability leave after giving birth. The changes in her body are real—and stressful. She shouldn't plan to be back at work in two weeks.

Can a new mother get six weeks of leave? Usually she can, though the amount of leave is not legally mandated. The Pregnancy Discrimination Act of 1978 requires employers to treat pregnancy-related disabilities on an equal basis with all other medical conditions. You have a right to be reinstated in your old job, if such reinstatements are company policy for other types of disability leaves. Nonetheless, your job may still be abolished in your absence. Maternity leave is no protection against layoffs if your company is in trouble, or if they wanted you to leave anyway.

In many states, state disability insurance covers six weeks of maternity leave. Employees of the federal government do not get state-provided leave and must use their own sick-leave and vacation to take time off. Some employers will supplement state disability payments until the combined payment is 50 or 75 percent of the employee's base pay. Other employers will not do this. Some very small companies may not subscribe to some states' disability plans. As you can see, there is immense variation in available maternity benefits, depending on what state you live in and your employer's policies. To assess your own situation, check first with your employer and then with your state office of unemployment insurance or disability benefits. This is usually listed in the phone book under State Offices—Employment Development or State Offices—Disability Insurance.

After you have learned about the benefits that may be coming to you, how should you financially prepare for the first few weeks of your baby's life? The following checklist will be helpful.

- Plan to take eight weeks off work.
- Find out what maternity-leave benefits your employer and your state offer.
- Put together a financial plan for expected expenses and sources of income.

First, be conservative: Expect to spend two weeks off work before you deliver and six weeks afterwards for recovery. It will take your body that long to get back to normal after pregnancy and labor, and most employers recognize this as "standard" leave time. Unless your employer's business is headed for layoffs, you should probably have no difficulty arranging to get your own job back at the end of this period.

Next, explore your options. Are you eligible for state

disability insurance? If you are, how much are you eligible for, and how do you apply? Rules for government programs can be tricky. One woman lost a full week's disability pay by working on a Monday. Usually there is a waiting period before disability payments start. Do you have company sick leave saved up to pay you during the waiting period? Will your company pay any supplementary benefits? If so, how much and for how long?

Disability before and after birth may come out of separate accounts. One woman was sure she had a total of six weeks of maternity leave, so she was quite upset when her doctor ordered her to stop work and rest in bed four weeks before her due date. "I thought 'Oh, no! Now I'll only have two weeks off to be with the baby.' But actually, I had six weeks off after the birth anyway. The time off the doctor ordered before the birth didn't come out of my maternity disability, which still started after the birth. It was very confusing."

Third, calculate how much money you will have coming in—from sick-leave pay, disability, and supplementary disability (if your employer has this). Add in your husband's pay. Make sure that you can pay the rent or mortgage, any car payments, and food expenses for those two months. If you can't meet these expenses from the income you will have, try to save money during your pregnancy to prepare.

The purpose of this planning is to assure that your first few weeks with the baby will be relatively untroubled by looming financial disasters. But as one woman said, "I don't know how we did it—with mirrors, I guess—but it all worked out." Two months isn't actually very long.

Planning for an Extended Leave

Some women reading this before they have a baby will assume that they don't have to read further. They will simply go back to work at four weeks, six weeks, or whenever. But be advised: Many women quit work altogether or go back only half-time. Others decide that they want a six-month leave of absence. Still others go back full-time but wish they could have taken more time off.

Of course, there may well be those mothers who go back to work after two weeks and love it. In interviewing for this book, we could not locate such women. The more common experience seems to be that women who go back to full-time jobs after only a few weeks wish that they didn't have to do so. They would prefer more time to rest, if nothing else. Plan for a longer leave, if at all possible. If you plan for a six-month leave or for six months half-time, you can always decide to go back full-time sooner, if you want to. Unfortunately, the reverse is not always true. Try to arrange for some flexibility for yourself.

Of course, not everyone can work part-time for a few months. For some women, especially single mothers, it may be very difficult to take any substantial amount of time off. Other women may be concerned that asking for extended leave will show lack of commitment to their jobs and derail their careers. They may also feel that if they are gone too long their employers will discover that they weren't really necessary.

What is a good length of time? Six weeks' leave is not really long enough. Many babies still don't know day from night at six weeks; many mothers are exhausted. Love between the mother and infant is beginning to grow, as the infant becomes more responsive and delivers his first fleeting smiles. Six weeks is no time at all.

On the other hand, at the end of six months most women are eager to get back to work, especially part-time. "I didn't want to be a housewife, a full-time servant," one woman said. "All the cooking, all the cleaning, always at home. That's not for me."

There is a definite loss of status, both outside the family and within the family, for women who give up their jobs. Few over-thirty mothers would choose to retire. They have a lot invested in their careers and they want the child to enrich their lives, not impoverish them (both financially and spiritually).

Having a baby while working means embarking on a

life of compromise. Leaving the baby with a sitter is a wrench . . . and a relief. How much of a wrench and how much of a relief depends, of course, on the unique personalities of mother and baby. The women who were happiest with their postpartum lives, however, seemed to have several things in common:

- They all used their stability, their job history, their professionalism to have a calm first few months of motherhood, and then they examined their further options.
- Despite later changes, they didn't rock the boat while they were pregnant. They negotiated successfully with their employers before the baby was born, being business-like about their upcoming change in circumstances. None of them planned to leave their jobs.
- They took between ten weeks and eight months of full-time leave and really enjoyed their babies.
- They went back to work part-time for the remainder of the first year.
- They all felt that it was easier to arrange the leave than they thought it would be. They had good, secure job histories and were confident of their company's investment in them as valuable employees. They continued to be in touch with things at the office during their leaves.
- They each seriously reassessed their careers when their babies were about six months old.
- Several of them changed jobs or started their own businesses within a year after the baby came, but they all had been very stable in their jobs during their pregnancies and in the early postpartum period.
- They had usually bought their homes several years before having a baby or else stayed in the same apartment after having the baby. In all cases, their mortgage or rent payments were within their capabilities, even on part-time pay.

- The ones who were married had emotionally supportive husbands.

In short, planning for a long leave is so dependent on
the mother's unique job and financial history that nobody
can really tell anyone else how to do it. Instead, here are
three women who did a good job of planning. Their experiences provide the best example.

The Accountant

"Actually, I never financially plan anything," says Jan.
"I'm not much of a planner. But when I knew I wanted to
have a baby, my lover and I got married. Then we took out
a loan to add on to his house, and I rented out my condo.
And I began saving sick leave at work (she worked at the
IRS) because government employees don't get any state
disability.

"By the time I had the baby, I had four months' sick
leave and vacation pay, and I then asked for four more
months' leave without pay, giving me eight months off
altogether. They gave it to me. I also asked for part-time
work for four months when I got back, to work only three
days a week. (I had decided not to work full-time the first
year.) They gave me the part-time work too. I was afraid,
with the bureaucracy, it would be hard to arrange all this,
but it was easy. I'd been there twelve years, and I guess
that counts, even in the government.

"The crazy part started when I went back after eight
months. I decided I just hated being there! I wanted to be
home more. So I added up my expenditures for the first
six months of the baby's life, simply by totalling up the
checks in my checkbook. Then I figured out what my husband earned for those six months, and I calculated what
I would have to earn to keep going. With my "target income" in mind, I began looking, and I found a job in a
medium-sized accounting firm in my area. They promised
me full-time work for tax time, and maybe one or two days
a week during the rest of the year. They paid me more per
day than the government had. I figured I could make it on

that, so I quit the IRS. I've really been happy! My daughter is two years old now, and I spend a lot of time with her."

A Single Mother

"I work as a nurse, and I used to live with a woman who was about my age (38) but who had had a child when she was twenty.

"I always wanted to have a child. I am not heterosexual. I spoke to my friends about having children, and most of them were in favor of artificial insemination. There is a women's health cooperative that provides that service. But I wanted to be able to let my child know who her father was. So I got pregnant by a friend.

"A few years ago, I had bought a house. When I decided to get pregnant, I figured that I would want to be home with the baby for a few months. I knew that I couldn't afford to do that and still make the house payments. When I got pregnant, I rented out the house and moved to a smaller place. I said to myself: Do I want this baby, or do I want to stay in this house? When I put it that way, it was very clear. I wanted a baby a lot more than I wanted the house.

"The move was good and bad. It was good because with the renter's payments to me plus my savings, I was able to take five months off to be with the baby. It was bad because my lover left me. The three of us in a small apartment were just too much for her.

"But everyone else has been great. My daughter's father comes by quite often, and I have a lot of friends who are very supportive. My dad is delighted; he always makes it clear that he supports my choices. My mother hasn't spoken to me in years, so what can I say about that? But my dad is very supportive, and even baby-sits on weekends.

"I took five months off work, full-time. Then I had to go back to work and get day care for my daughter. So I've stayed in the same apartment; the extra income from the house really helps with the child-care expenses. When she's bigger, though, I'll want to move back to the house. For now, it is all working out."

The Hospital Administrator

"I've been working for the same company for eight years, ever since it was founded. We do consultation and training in hospitals. I took ten weeks off full-time when I had Mary, but I called into the office a lot and stopped by and kept up with my projects. Then I went back to work half-time for about three months, and then 80 percent time. I feel I can leave at the stroke of five o'clock now without feeling guilty. Mary is almost a year old, but I'm not sure when I'll go to full-time; this is working out so well.

"I couldn't have done this in my twenties. Back then, I was working sixty to seventy hours a week—the company was really new, I was trying to prove myself. And nobody would have cared that much for me, to give me this sort of leave. Also, we've been in our house for six years, and our mortgage payments are very low. I don't know how younger women have babies, actually, with their big new house payments and nobody to be as understanding as my bosses have been."

FAMILY BARGAINING: WHATEVER HAPPENED TO THE WEEKEND SKI TRIPS?

Financial planning may include the employers, but it also includes the husband. Many two-career marriages are also two-checking-account marriages. Husband and wife may contribute equally to the shared payments (rent, groceries) while maintaining their own accounts (my car, my clothes, my money).

There are obvious problems with this system when a baby is involved. If the wife is off work for several months, how can she carry her end of the payments? Should she have to save up for her maternity leave, while he continues to have money available for a new ten-speed bike? In short, is the change in income status her problem, or is it a family problem?

Strangely enough, two people who have slept together for fifteen years may still have a great deal of trouble blending their checking accounts. That is just too much intimacy! It takes a new degree of trust, letting him have total access to your money. It takes a reassessment of the basis for the relationship, when you depend on his financial support. It is not easy.

Nobody said that parenthood was easy. The trouble is that it is hard in unexpected ways. Reaching into a family's financial life and giving advice is much harder than giving advice about their sex life. With sex, at least, the goals are clearly defined: good sex for all; only the method for achieving those goals is in doubt. With finances, it is different. The very goals are in doubt. A good time now versus saving for the future? An elegant house or a succession of late-model cars? Do children need music lessons and private schools, or is it just as good to have them in organized sports and public schools? Compatibility can become combativeness very easily.

With a child, financial arrangements will have to change, and this sort of change can be painful. There will be less money to spend on the adults and more joint decision-making about the remaining money. Each couple must work out individual solutions to this problem: It will undoubtedly be harder when the two partners have had separate checking accounts and expensive hobbies than when they always shared a checking account and were religious about saving money.

But we do have one suggestion that many parents have found helpful. Everybody needs some money to spend without asking someone else's permission. In short, everybody needs an allowance. This allowance should be very firmly fixed, and payable whether or not the person who gets it is earning money at that time. Even if the allowance is only five dollars a week, it is useful. Ten to twenty dollars a week is much better. Every wife or husband needs to be able to buy a record or go out to lunch with a friend without feeling guilty.

Try to give yourself some emotional breathing space by having as large a personal allowance as feasible. The availability of this small amount of money, to be spent totally at your discretion, can smooth negotiations about much larger issues.

Mother and father must realize, together, that there won't be weekend ski trips for a while. Nor will there be much discretionary money. Taking care of a baby is expensive.

But it has its rewards. Few parents would trade their children for all the ski trips and late-model cars in the world. Or for all the tea in China.

Single Mothers
by Choice

If the world were perfect, perhaps, there would be no single mothers. There wouldn't be fewer men than women in the thirty- to thirty-nine-year-old age group, because men wouldn't die younger. All men would be capable of being committed fathers, and the divorce courts and the lawyers specializing in collecting child support would be out of business. While we're describing what ought to be, let's not forget to ban war, hunger, and disease, also.

But it isn't a perfect world. For many women, when it comes to motherhood, the question is whether to be single mothers or not be mothers at all. Their childhood expectations (first you marry Mr. Right, then you buy a house with some rosebushes, then you have a baby) no longer apply. And it becomes clear that a woman needn't be married and in charge of some hybrid tea roses in order to be a good mother.

There is no doubt that single women who are mothers by choice have a more difficult life in some ways. All the financial responsibility, all the arrangements, all the caring fall on one set of shoulders. In interviewing women for this chapter, we expected to talk to many whose shoulders were stooped under the burden.

Instead we found women delighted with their motherhood. After having given up on the possibility for years, they then, in their thirties, found the courage to say, "This is what I want." As a group, they were far more positive, cheerful, and pleased with themselves and their children than the average divorced woman was. They were members of single-mothers groups, and both the lesbian and heterosexual women had found ways to involve men in their parenting. They were having problems, but they were also finding solutions.

SINGLE MOTHERS BY CHOICE OR CHANCE

There are many roads to single motherhood, and more and more women are taking them. Some women discover they are pregnant unintentionally and then choose birth and motherhood instead of abortion. Others want to be mothers but don't want to marry their lover, because he is not committed to fatherhood. Some are deliberately choosing to bear children alone, going to a sperm bank and paying for donor insemination. Others are lesbian women, and still others find themselves single mothers after becoming divorced or widowed.

As a matter of fact, so many roads lead to "single woman, head of household" that in 1984 fully 25 percent of the children in this country were living in single-parent families. Fifty percent of black children were living with only one parent, as were 20 percent of white children. Approximately nineteen out of twenty single-parent families were headed by a woman. Though there are men with custody of their children, for a first approximation, the terms *single parent* and *single mother* can be used interchangeably.

Divorced women head by far the largest group of single-parent households. The average duration of a marriage in the United States is 9.4 years, which is long enough to have a set of children but not long enough to raise them. Current estimates are that 50 percent of the children born in the late '70s will face the divorce of their parents before the children are sixteen.

The next-largest group of single mothers is young women. Many teen-age pregnancies end in abortion, but the young women who choose to bear the baby also usually choose to keep it. In 1978, according to the Guttmacher Institute, 96 percent of all unwed teen-agers who gave birth kept the baby.

Comparatively few older women have babies out of wedlock, but the trend is growing. Approximately 10 percent of the babies born to women thirty to thirty-nine years of age are born out of wedlock.

The path a single mother takes is not an easy one. It can be lonely. If a child is sick, there may be nobody to share her anxiety. When a child wins a sports trophy or a school honor, who but the mother is there to care?

And single mothers are often poor. "If mothers just had more money, a great many of their problems would vanish," says Debby Lee, a single mother, and director of San Francisco's Early Single Parenting Project. Ms. Lee has led many support groups for single parents. As she explains: "Even women who are not poor when they become single parents are often impoverished by motherhood. Day-care and child-rearing expenses come out of a woman's salary, which, on the average, is only 40 percent of a man's. Even those in the upper economic echelon of single mothers are comparatively poor. Say there's a well-off single mother with a good job. Her own major problem may not be poverty. But if you compare her with a well-paid married woman who also has a working husband, you have to admit . . . relatively, she's poor."

Nevertheless, women in their thirties are choosing to be single mothers. The focus of this chapter is on the women who make that choice. Who are they, and why do they choose the single-parent option? And an even more important question: How do they make it work?

Getting to Yes

Teen-age women have "accidents." Married women have "accidents." When an older unmarried woman carries a baby to term, it is rarely an accident. She has made a choice.

Many older single women have used birth control successfully for fifteen years. Many have had previous abortions. Their decision to become a mother *this time* rests on the same two motivating factors that force the older married woman into the decision-making mode. First, biologically, it is now or never for motherhood; you can't keep thinking about it through an endless series of tomorrows. Second, with increased maturity you are aware that there is no such thing as a perfect time or situation for motherhood.

Single motherhood is not the first choice for most educated, middle-class women. Few women, when they were adolescent girls, dreamed about raising a baby alone. But many things can happen between adolescence and the age of thirty. Older women who want to be mothers have learned that life is not a fairly tale, furnished with perfect husband and home.

While interviewing single women who were mothers by choice, one theme reappeared over and over: the determination to be mothers. Those who were pregnant when interviewed were delighted with their pregnancies. Indeed, on these subjects they showed much less ambivalence than the average married woman did. The pregnant married women seemed to spend more energy worrying about how it was all going to work. Most of the single women were truly pleased to be fulfilling a life goal that they had almost given up on achieving. Their attitude was often much more positive.

These positive attitudes and the various ways the women managed to make single motherhood work for them are reflected in the case histories below. (Also see the single mother's story in Chapter 3 on financial planning.) It seems worthwhile to let the women themselves speak before we draw conclusions about how to make single motherhood successful.

Woman on Welfare

"My doctor told me that I could never get pregnant, because I had endometriosis. He suggested that taking the birth-control pill would hold my disease in check. But I didn't want to take the pill; I wanted to have a baby. So I went off the pill, and the miracle happened.

"I was ecstatic! I was a graduate student and a teaching assistant, and I told all my students. Several women said to me that they'd never heard anyone in a professional position speak so positively about being pregnant, that I had really been inspiring. Well, I felt inspired, every day. Breaking up with my lover when I was four months along was traumatic, but I was basically still so happy to be pregnant.

"After the baby was born, I had the same problem 98 percent of single mothers have: how to have time to take care of my baby and also earn enough to support myself. Society has these boxes: One is labeled 'wage-earner' and the other is labeled 'nurturer.' Both are supposed to be full-time positions. Frankly, it was a problem I didn't solve for the first eighteen months. Or rather, I solved it by going on welfare. Actually, welfare doesn't pay enough to live on: If I hadn't had friends helping me, I don't know what I would have done. When my son was eighteen months old, I felt he was old enough for some day care, and I got a job.

"It is surprisingly hard to get off welfare. For one thing, welfare comes with a sort of medical coverage; here in California it's called Medi-Cal. As soon as you go to work, you lose that Medi-Cal. If you work at the average minimum-wage job, you don't get any insurance benefits. So welfare is actually safer, in terms of having medical coverage for the baby. After a while, I found a part-time job in a social service agency that did have a decent benefits plan. I made sure to work enough hours to qualify for the medical coverage. Even a part-time professional job pays more than welfare, so the money was okay.

"Another major difficulty was arranging for child care while I wasn't working. It is really hard to be with a baby twenty-four hours a day, never to have anyone who will take him for a few minutes. You can go crazy. And of course, while I was on welfare, I couldn't pay for a baby-sitter.

"Luckily, I have a lot of friends who really like children. Now that my son is nine, he chooses to spend much of his time at friends' houses. That really started when he was small, when I would arrange for various people to enjoy his company for a while, while I took a break.

"And I really mean 'enjoy his company.' He's a gift and a treasure, and why shouldn't other people have a chance to appreciate and love him? There are a lot of people who like children, despite what you hear. I feel like he's a resource to share, not a burden to impose. And it has worked out well. It saved my sanity when he was a baby, and he has plenty of friends now. I'm working full-time, and we're both happy. It's worthwhile to have a positive attitude."

Day-Care Dilemma

(Note: The following woman did not choose to be a single mother; her husband left her two weeks before the birth. Yet her story highlights some of the problems of single parenthood very clearly. She was caught in a trap: a single parent from the birth of the child but with many decisions, such as where to live and where to work, made as a married woman.)

"I had been married for sixteen years when I got pregnant. I wanted children, but my husband didn't want any. When I was two weeks from delivery, he left me.

"I had arranged to go back to work part-time after the baby was born. Well, that was out of the question. I had to go back full-time when she was eight weeks old. And the trouble I had with day care! Really, it's like a soap opera. The first problem was: Where should the day care be? I work thirty miles from home, so should the day-care person be near my home or near my work?

"The first one I chose was near my work. She always made me pay cash in advance, which should have worried me, but she was very nice, and there were several other children going there, including the daughter of one of my friends. Well, one Monday we learned she had skipped town over the weekend.

"The next person I chose was also very sweet but turned out to be an alcoholic. I was terrified. First, that I'd left my daughter with her, and second, that I was without day care again. This time I found someone good, but she could do it for only one month, because her day-care home was technically 'full' and she couldn't take any more children.

"Finally, I found someone really good, near my home. It seems to be working very well. But my daughter had four day-care homes in less than five months, which can't be good. Also, day care near home really has some drawbacks. I have to leave work by five on the dot or I'll be late picking her up. I'm not used to that.

"Also, there was so much pain when my husband left. I had to get used to this rejection. I spent days thinking: If he was going to leave me, why didn't he do it ten years ago, so I could have married someone else and had babies and lived happily ever after? But on the other hand, I'm glad I'm old enough to be established in my career and mature enough to be a single parent."

The Adoptive Mother

"At forty-two, I was living with a man who was ambivalent about having a baby. I tried to get pregnant by him, but I had fertility problems. I really was obsessed with babies. I got on a foster parents list, to sort of 'try out' parenthood.

"As a foster parent, I took care of a baby for three weeks. I loved being around that baby! I knew then that having a child was terribly important to me, much more important than living with my lover. We broke up about six months after my foster parenting experience.

"Meanwhile, I told all my friends that I wanted to adopt. Many of my friends are social workers. Three months after I had moved out on my own, a friend called. Would I care to meet a young couple who were planning to give up their baby when it was born? I met them the next day. Seven days after the interview she had the baby, and three days later I brought home my little girl.

"Once a year, I write the birth mother and the father. Writing is part of the terms of the 'private adoption,' but I also feel good about doing it. They are real people to me. They chose me. I want to let them know she's happy.

"I didn't have much time to plan. One week! But I have such wonderful friends! People came over with baby clothes, with a crib—with everything. A friend helped me find good day care. I was only working half-time, so I had a lot of time with the baby. I also rented a room to a student, who does some child care and housework for me.

"I worked half-time till Janet was six months old. Then I worked four days a week, because I needed the money. When she was a year old I needed more money, so I went back full-time.

"I felt, and I still feel, that my life has just gotten better and better since I adopted Janet. She is such a happy, outgoing child, a miracle. I feel I can do anything, because I could do this. Now I feel I can look at men differently. I'm seeing a very kind and generous and loving man right now. We're looking toward a permanent relationship.

"Life has just gotten better and better, ever since I adopted my little girl."

SPECIAL CHALLENGES OF SINGLE MOTHERHOOD

As one single mother pointed out to members of her support group, "I have a photo album full of pictures of my son, but no pictures of both of us. There is nobody around to take those pictures." From society's point of view, the older single mother and her problems are as invisible as she is in her child's pictures.

Some of the concerns of the single-mother-by-choice are common to all working mothers; others are unique.

"Arranging" for a Baby

For married couples, the first step in arranging for a baby is usually simple, unless there is a fertility problem. For a single woman, there are too many choices.

Some single women face an after-the-fact choice. They become pregnant as a consequence of birth-control failure or their own ambivalence about continuing to use birth control. Then they must choose between pregnancy and abortion. For the over-thirty woman, pregnancy is often her choice. She may feel that this is her last chance to have a baby.

Other women deliberately choose to have a child and are then faced with a variety of choices on how to get pregnant. A woman's choices range from artificial insemination (the ultimate in father uninvolvement) through the biological parents living together in a committed manner and coparenting (marriage without benefit of state license). There is also the possibility of adoption.

Adoption is undoubtedly the hardest. There is a shortage of "perfect" adoptable babies (healthy newborns), and so the single mother will almost certainly not be able to adopt such a child—unless she goes through private placement, as did the adoptive mother described earlier. In many private adoptions, the adoptive mother stays in touch with the biological mother, writing letters about the child's progress. As one such single mother put it, "I had to offer something special. Or else why would any biological mother pick me, instead of Mr. and Mrs. Upper-Middle-Class America?"

For many women, bearing the child themselves is an important part of being a mother. Some find the question of how to get pregnant a fairly easy one, the answers ranging from "with a loving boyfriend" to "a one-night stand." Both of these methods have their drawbacks. The loving boyfriend may not want to be a father, or he may become an overinvolved and unwelcome visitor later in the child's life. The one-night stand may leave the mother very embarrassed at the child's questions later. "I'd hate to have to tell my child that I couldn't remember his father's name or face," said one mother.

None of the women interviewed for this book actually chose the singles-bar route. They weren't willing to start their adventure in commitment and love with an experience so lacking in both. Women who got pregnant by men they knew, even if the men weren't willing to coparent, seemed to feel content with their decision.

Donor insemination, the third option, has some advantages over the singles bar. If nothing else, the donor center screens the applicants, so donor insemination is less likely to transmit disease. It is also the method of choice for some (but not all) lesbian women. Nonetheless, any time you get involved with a technological fix to a human problem, you introduce another set of complications: dealing with the guardians of the technology. Many doctors will not artificially inseminate a single woman. A woman must find a cooperative doctor or a feminist health group in order to make this method work. Women who choose this method are also concerned with what to tell the child about his or her heritage.

For some women, donor insemination can eliminate many personal obstacles that might otherwise seem insuperable. One woman chose donor insemination shortly after breaking up with a long-term boyfriend. "I had some fertility problems," she said, "and I didn't want to have to start off my next relationship with a discussion of our medical histories."

Practical Problems to Resolve While Pregnant

Once the baby is on the way, through either pregnancy or adoption, the first problem is financial. If the single mother is going to have any time off to be with her baby, she has to carefully plan her self-support. A married couple may be able to drop from two incomes to one income for a few months, but a single mother may have a hard time dropping from one income to none.

We found, however, in interviewing for this book, that the single mothers did a better job of financial planning than most of the married couples had. They knew they had only themselves to rely upon, so they saved up, moved other people into their home to share the expenses, or else arranged for day care with a relative. Single mothers were often more flexible than were married couples. While the couples, as a group, were concerned about keeping up their standard of living, some single mothers were even willing to go on welfare if it helped them achieve their goals of mothering. Note, however, that health insurance needs are virtually the same for both married and single mothers (Chapter 3 on financial planning contains information on this important topic).

One area in which married women have the edge over the single mother is in announcing their pregnancy. A pregnant married woman has society's approval, even if her career progress is somewhat jeopardized. Attitudes toward a pregnant unmarried woman range from disapproval (that woman sinned!) through pity for her plight. She won't be driven out into a blizzard, but simple acceptance of her condition may be very hard to come by, even in this enlightened age. The double standard is alive and well and living in your office.

Many women have said that not giving much information is the best way to handle questions. Answering questions just leads to more questions, as they teach soldiers who are likely to be captured by the enemy; "Just give them your name, rank, and serial number." With this in mind, just tell them that you are glad to be pregnant, what your due date is, and how long you expect to be off work. A coworker doesn't have the right or need to know who the father is or what your living arrangements will be. A simple "That's a personal question" can often work wonders.

A third problem that single mothers face is the possibility of giving birth alone. As we say in Chapter 7, a helpful and encouraging labor partner can make the labor a lot easier on the mother. After delivery, women with labor coaches often feel more alert and ready to cuddle the baby. It is not required that the labor coach be the baby's father.

One lesbian mother gave birth with three coaches and a photographer in attendance. "It was me and my army," she jokes. Some women have had their sisters there; others have friends who are very pleased to help out. Being involved in a birth is very exciting. Many people would consider it an honor rather than an imposition to be asked to be your labor coach.

Postpartum: The Pressures of an Early Return to Work

A single mother will find that while many people will offer emotional support, it will be up to her to undertake her own financial support. That often means an early return to work. It seems that the rich and the poor manage this part of motherhood more easily: They don't go back to work early and full time.

There are single mothers (often doctors, psychologists, or entrepeneurs) who are so well paid that they need only go back to work part time. These women have a lot of time to spend with their children. This is an advantage of making over forty dollars an hour.

There are other single mothers who have low incomes but still only work part time. They generally share living arrangements and child care with other people, so that the group acts as an extended family. These mothers also can spend a lot of time with their children. This is an advantage of being unconventional.

Single mothers who are neither rich nor unconventional face the necessity of an early return to work. No work—no money, period. These mothers face the same problems of finding child care that married women face (see Chapter 10 on choosing day care), but without the twin salaries to pay for it. As Debby Lee said, "Single mothers' biggest problem is poverty." This is especially true for the middle-class woman hoping to keep a middle-class lifestyle.

In all this, the one major advantage that a single mother has over a married woman is that she has only her own and her child's needs to consider. She can set her own priorities. If she is rich, she can spend her money buying free time for herself, rather than making expensive mortgage payments. If she isn't, she can still make her own decisions about her temporary lifestyle.

Some single-mothers-by-choice are willing to follow their original nonstandard choice with some further unusual decisions. This allows them more flexibility, and they seem to have less upheaval in their day-to-day lives.

Home with Baby: Somebody Give Me a Break!

"Ironically, as a result of my unconventional behavior I was forced into domestic arrangements that were far more rigid than those of women in more conventional households. I had to be more efficient, for one thing, because there was no one else around to say, 'I'll do the dishes, honey; you must be tired.' It has taken me nearly five years of practice to learn to control the feeling of hysteria that used to come over me whenever the door closed on Amy and her baby-sitter, who were off to the park for two precious hours (eight dollars). Should I wash my hair or write a lecture or go shopping or try to sleep? Is it worth a dollar to sit staring at the wall for fifteen minutes, which is what I really *want* to do?" This is how Phyllis Mack, a professor, describes her life as a single mother in an article in *Ms.* magazine. According to Debby MacIntosh, another single mother: "They say that when you have the time, you don't have the money, and when you have the money, you don't have the time. When you're a single parent, it's not one or the other, it's neither."

"Buying time" is a phrase that every single mother understands, because so often any break from the baby has to be paid for. Many women are stunned at the amount of money they spend for child care. It is really worth planning ahead to avoid some of this expense.

For example, can you share your living arrangements with another single parent, your lover, or a student who needs a place to stay in return for baby-sitting ten hours a week? Can you join a single-parents support group and make informal arrangements with another mother ("I'll take them Tuesday nights, you take them Thursday")? Can you arrange with your mother or sister to take the baby for a few hours each weekend? Explore your own options. A single mother will probably be spending a lot of money on child care in order to work. She should try to arrange for some free time for herself in a less expensive manner.

How well these informal arrangements work out depends on your situation (a sister in town can be a great help), but it also depends on your attitude. If you feel that taking care of the child is an awful thing to ask of anyone else, if you are covered with guilt about your need to finish an occasional meal in peace, it may be hard to make these arrangements. If you see your child as a beautiful resource to be shared, a happy person that others will just naturally want to spend some time with, informal arrangements tend to come more easily. As the first mother interviewed in this chapter noted, "It is worthwhile to have a positive attitude."

The Man in Your Child's Life

The great benefits that children can derive from their fathers are described in the next chapter. What does that mean for single mothers? What if daddy is not around?

A woman raising a child alone should realize that the man in her child's life doesn't have to be the child's father. The lesbian mother described above encouraged her own father to baby-sit: Grandfathers can be great for children. Another single mother chose to rent part of her house to a married couple who had a small child. Many men really do like children, and they are as much of a resource as your women friends and relatives.

And don't forget the baby's father. He may not want complete, traditional involvement, but he often has a certain level of caring. His commitment may not be adequate for a marriage, but it can be vastly beneficial to the child.

Again, in many ways single mothers have more leeway than married women, not less. A married woman whose husband is not very interested in the baby may see only one choice ahead: nagging him to do his part. A single-by-choice mother can be more accepting of the father's lack of involvement. She can arrange for the child to spend Saturday afternoons with her married brother, or she can move in with a man who is interested in coparenting. As Deva Lowenthal said in an article in the *Northern California Jewish Bulletin:* "You learn that you can't rely on FOB (father of baby)—a painful lesson divorced women learn much later."

Many fathers drift in and out of their children's lives. Single mothers are often rather philosophical about the man's role. They are not too surprised if he is helpful for a few months after the birth, then drifts away and then returns in a couple of years. On the other hand, a married woman would be filled with rancor at such a father. Single mothers are often more cynical about the biological father, but they are also less angry at him. This attitude cannot help but enhance the child's relationship with his father. To some extent, single women have learned to coparent with imperfect men.

A SINGLE MOTHER'S PRIMER

Single mothers choose a tough and demanding life. With love and planning, however, it can be a very satisfying one.

Many children (11 million as of this writing) are living in single-parent households. Only a very small fraction of those children were brought into the world (or adopted) by an older single woman who expected to raise the child alone. Nevertheless, those who have chosen to be single mothers often have a special brand of guilt. They are single parents by choice. If anything goes wrong, it must be all their fault.

Anybody who raises children has lots of opportunities for things to go wrong, no matter how many parents are in the family. Once again we must stress that nobody on this Earth does parenthood "right." Everybody is living a first approximation to the life he or she wants to lead. There is no particular reason for a single mother to feel guilty. Overwhelmed on occasion, yes. Guilty, no.

Why should a woman who truly wanted a child and is doing everything she can to raise that child well feel guilty? Because she has to work? According to government statistics, 48 percent of preschool children had working mothers; those mothers weren't all single. Is she guilty because she hasn't provided her children with a man around the house? Since the average length of a marriage is nine years nowadays, marriage certainly doesn't provide children any guarantees of having a loving and attentive father.

Older single mothers are usually resourceful people. They may not have much financial security, but they can often be extremely creative in making use of what is available to them. They make a real effort to have friends involved with their children. Studies of infant-mother interactions often show the mother interacting less with the infant when the father is around. Another parent can be distracting, as well as helpful.

The single mothers who are genuinely happy with their role and relaxed with their children have several things in common.

- They see their choice as positive ("something I wanted to do and did") rather than guilt-provoking ("something I managed to do, but not the way it should be done").

- They deliberately (or naturally) set up large, rather free-form support networks. They often have unconventional friends who sometimes keep unconventional hours, and who are really ready to pitch in during a crisis. To a certain extent, these women have reinvented the extended family, without the constraints of biological kinship or the in-fighting of communes. Many participate in single-mother support groups as part of this process.

• They have made a careful choice of where and how to live. Single motherhood in a single house in suburbia is very difficult. Shared housing often works better. Motherhood on your own also seems to be easier in cities or near universities, or anywhere that people aren't all paired up. Also, convenience of home to work and work to day care is very important. The single mother cannot afford the time, money, or schedule inflexibility of a long commute.

• They think positively and have confidence in their ultimate ability to raise their children. That is not the same as saying there are no moments of panic or days of despair. There are. As one woman said, "There are days when I'd trade everything, feminism included, for a man around the house." Nevertheless, the successful single mothers see themselves as parents who are able to solve problems with and for their kids.

• They have arranged emotional support for themselves during pregnancy and labor and for the first months home with the baby. (In the reference section, we list some nationwide single-mothers' resource centers.) While these women are active in single-mother support groups, they also have men in their lives and in their children's lives.

• They are willing to give themselves credit. As Debby Lee, director of the Early Single Parenting Project says, "Single motherhood is work. It isn't visible work: Nobody says what a great job you're doing, nobody pays you to do it. There is nobody there but yourself and the child when you are working. But raising a child is hard work, and I always tell women to give themselves some credit for it."

If you find yourself pregnant unintentionally, really think about whether you want to do this. The combination of child-care expenses and time constraints and parental responsibility can be very stressful. Read Chapter 6 for help in making your decision.

If you do decide to be a single mother, it is most practical to get pregnant by someone you know. Adoption can be difficult to arrange, and donor insemination or one-night stands can be hard to explain to a child. A father who is known but isn't around much will give the child a context rather similar to that of about half the kids at school.

Also, arrange for some emotional support for yourself during pregnancy. Ask a friend or relative to be your labor coach. And arrange for some child-care support for yourself after you have the baby.

Above all, forgive yourself for your errors. Do you think every married woman is a perfect mother? Is a wedding band that magical? You and your child will probably do just fine.

Fathering the Working Family*

In Chapter 1, we described the "double image" facing modern women who are deciding about motherhood. Modern men approaching fatherhood are faced with a similar double image. The first ideal is that of the "good provider": success on the job, long hours, and the search for excellence. The second ideal is the egalitarian helper: the sensitive, sharing man, who is emotionally supportive to his wife and who cooks and helps with the baby.

But there aren't that many hours in the day. If being a good provider means working twelve-hour days, and being a sensitive husband means doing most of the baby care when home, that doesn't leave much time to sleep.

How to resolve these conflicting demands? Today's father cannot usually find guidance in his own past. Unlike

---

*A note to the reader: While this book as a whole has been addressed to women, this chapter should be read by both the parents-to-be. Many of the "helpful hint" lists, for example, are addressed directly to fathers.

his own father, who probably paced the hospital waiting room at his son's birth, the modern father expects to assist with his wife's labor. He is also willing to change diapers. His wife is going back to work in a few weeks or months. But he has no firm model in his head for what this new type of fatherhood involves, once he's past the delivery room. When you're an explorer, there aren't any signposts.

A brief view of fatherhood from a biological and cross-cultural perspective will show why the signposts are missing. After that, we will hear from the older fathers of this generation: what they feel, how they act, and what they can best do for the family.

BIOLOGICAL AND CULTURAL FATHERHOOD

Biology itself, male sexual functioning, provides no guide to fatherhood. Biologically complete fatherhood can involve a commitment of fewer than five minutes. Millions of men have fathered children without ever knowing that they had done so. And even when men know they are fathers, a sense of obligation to woman and child is not automatic.

After the first few minutes, fatherhood is less of a biological fact than a cultural expectation, and the role of the father is one of the most free-floating variables in anthropological literature. Mothers universally bear and nurse infants, but fatherhood has no such built-in guideposts.

Take the father's role in pregnancy. In many societies, including our own, the husband of a pregnant woman has no clearly defined role. In other groups, however, this is not so. Among the Arapesh, a tribe in Papuan New Guinea, the father must "grow" the baby with contributions of semen. He is expected to have vigorous intercourse with his wife as often as possible during the first months of pregnancy. Other tribes expect the man to observe certain food taboos while his wife is pregnant, or to refrain from hunting certain animals.

After the baby is born, the fathers' roles vary again. Among the Lesu of Melanesia, men will often play with a baby or small child for hours. On the other hand, Rwala Bedouin fathers studiously ignore all children younger than five. Among the Rwala, the father's first major duty to his children is to circumcise his son when the boy is about five years old.

And then there are the matrilineal societies in which the father spends little time with his own children but helps raise his sister's children. And the societies where men live in separate houses (men's houses) and only visit the women's dwellings. Children live with the women until the boys are old enough to join their fathers in the men's houses.

In the Western world, many occupations require men to be absent from their families for months or years at a time. Men are soldiers, sailors, oil-field workers at remote sites. Sending money home is essential to these men's fatherhood: Helping to raise the children is simply not possible. For these men, there can be no double image of provider versus helper. Provider is the only role they can fill.

Most of the men reading this chapter don't have such a straightforward resolution of the provider-versus-helper dilemma. They must find their fatherhood balance in a more complex manner. Some understanding of the strains of the dual role, along with some information on how to be a successful (in every sense of the word) modern father can be helpful. The information that follows has come from psychological research and from interviews with fathers themselves.

FATHERS OF THE WESTERN WORLD

The First Nine Months of Fatherhood

Being pregnant is a family stress, not just a change in maternal physiology. Men feel they must be emotionally supportive at home and very much business-as-usual at the office. Their own feelings of uncertainty and fear are usually suppressed. After all, the woman has problems of her own; no use burdening her with his worries.

The trouble with suppressing feelings is that it doesn't work. Studies have shown that many fathers-to-be have extremely empathetic reactions to their wife's condition. For example, many men gain weight during their wife's pregnancy. They have digestive upsets that mimic morning sickness. They feel irritable. "I was crabby with everyone—except my wife," one man said.

Empathy reactions are common enough in pregnant fathers to have a technical name: couvade symptoms. *Couvade* comes from the French word for "cover" or "hatch," as if the father were helping to hatch the child.

The old joke says, "We've never lost a father yet." That joke is a put-down of fathers, devaluing their natural and normal anxiety. One man described his feelings of frustration at not being able to help his wife more. "We made the decision together that this was the time to have a child. But then, after she got pregnant, I realized that it was all happening in her body, not mine. I know, that's obvious, but have you ever noticed how many men say 'when *we* got pregnant'? But believe me, *she* gets pregnant. I was expecting to feel excited, but actually I was worried. I also felt left out, though I couldn't tell her that."

Besides the inability to share the wife's pregnancy, there may also be other frustrations. This is especially true if the couple does not, or cannot, have sexual relations for a large portion of the pregnancy. "I wasn't getting my needs met," one husband said. "And I couldn't even say anything about it. I mean, I felt embarrassed to tell her how I felt."

Many men are also concerned about their ability to be a good father. The father-to-be begins to think about his own father—how the older man was a good father or how he failed. Old conflicts sleeping since adolescence may well resurface in his mind. Unfortunately, where a woman might talk to a friend about her relationship with her mother, men are often more reticent. But working through what "fathering" means, from a new perspective, is an important task in a man's maturation.

Some men get very worried about finances while their wives are pregnant. Quite a few even change jobs. (Hopefully, a man who changes jobs while his wife is pregnant has carefully reviewed the insurance situation discussed in Chapter 3.) In interviewing for this book, we met a freelancer who joined a large company (for more security) when his wife got pregnant, and we met a lawyer who struck out on his own in the hopes of raising his income. Most men don't change jobs, but they all seem to worry. The "good provider" image becomes especially vivid at this time, particularly if the wife is planning to take a long maternity leave.

These are the problems, but what are the solutions? The only solution is to realize that pregnancy is a strain on the father as well as the mother. He needs a defined role, and he needs someone to talk to. Let's take the couvade symptoms as an example.

Jacqueline Clinton studied the couvade phenomenon. (Her work was reported in an article by Joy Lewis.) She found that expectant fathers who have some outward expression of their change in status find that they can relieve the emotional strain. In this sense, tribes with food taboos for the father-to-be—"I can't eat that, she's pregnant"—have come up with an excellent way to let the man acknowledge his special state and feel he is doing something to help his wife.

Food taboos wouldn't work in the Western world, though we did interview one father who invented his own taboo by giving up smoking. But childbirth education classes can be a big help. In these classes, the father-to-be learns practical ways to help his wife prepare for the birth. He meets other men going through the same experience. Giving a man an acceptable way to get involved with the pregnancy is one of the major benefits of the childbirth education classes.

The husband also needs some acknowledgment of his concerns by his wife. Sexual needs are among the easiest to deal with. (See Chapter 7, where we discuss intercourse during pregnancy.) Some deprivations are not necessary.

Communication links between the expectant parents are more complicated, and they take more work. Over and over, fathers we interviewed explained how they could not reveal their negative feelings or their fears to their wives. In this case, the wife must take some initiative, bring up issues, be willing to listen. And that support needs to be reciprocated.

Pregnancy, like parenthood, requires sharing.

Tips for Pregnant Fathers

▶ Don't be ashamed of your empathy reactions to the pregnancy. It isn't weird, it's natural. Relax, and don't worry if you both feel a little under the weather.

▶ Allow your wife to pamper you on occasion. You need it.

▶ Don't worry too much about money. Read Chapter 3 and do what you can to prepare. But remember, it isn't necessary to be a millionaire to be a good father.

▶ Love each other, both physically and emotionally. You are on a great adventure together. Try to enjoy it.

The Father of an Infant

After pregnancy comes birth, and then the child comes home from the hospital. One man describes how he felt when he first brought his wife and baby home.

"When I drove to the hospital door, they brought my

wife over to the car in a wheelchair. The nurse helped her into the car, and then she handed her the baby. I remember thinking, 'My god, what have I let myself in for? I'm really responsible for these people now. My wife can't help me; she's even in a wheelchair. *What am I going to do?*' "

Talking to new fathers seems to guarantee talk about responsibility. It comes as a shock, especially to older men, how incredibly dependent a baby is and how much their wives have become dependent upon them. "Responsibility," "the breadwinner," "a good provider"—all the issues they thought they had certainly resolved are back again. It is a new and somewhat upsetting view of what it means to be an adult male, having relatively helpless people depending on you.

But breadwinning is only part of the problem for the modern father. He is also struggling with the definition of half the housework and baby care. "I'll bet every older father in America is going through the same thing," one man said. "My wife says that I don't do half the baby care. I know I don't. I do all the grocery shopping, I cook many of the meals, I change diapers. But I'm gone all day, and I don't do half the baby care even when I'm home. And it seems that she is always mad at me about it."

While she is jealous of his freedom from baby care, he may be jealous of her involvement with the baby. This jealousy takes many forms. "Let's face it, she just doesn't have much time for me or my concerns anymore," another man said. "I guess it is natural, but I don't have to like it."

Others are envious of their wife's freedom to stay home. "She was so involved with the baby, so attuned to him," said one father. "Meanwhile, I was juggling the bills, and frankly, we were getting behind. She was looking for a job with flexible hours, and I was very supportive of her desire to be with the baby. At least I said I was very supportive. But when the baby was ten months old, I began to feel that she was stalling, looking for the perfect situation, that she didn't care whether the family went under financially, as long as she could stay home and play with the baby."

Being the father of a baby is stressful, especially for

the older man. Old patterns of living, of getting attention, of dealing with finances are interrupted, changed forever, and they must be reformulated. This takes time and patience and a lot of communicating. Since men are often ashamed of their feelings ("I can't be jealous of a baby; I should be a better provider"), it is usually up to the woman to begin the communication process.

Both husband and wife should keep in mind that there is no fifty-fifty solution to baby care. Except in homes where there is complete role reversal (mother goes back to work and father stays home), men simply do not take over half the child care in the first few months. (Dividing the work between husband and wife is discussed in Chapter 8; here we are really concentrating on the father.)

Though the father cannot do half the work, he must take on some of it. If all Dad does is play with the baby after dinner, it won't be enough to keep the household going. The man is going to have to do some diapering, some cuddling, and some bathing, or, frankly, the house (and the mother) will probably collapse.

While a man's involvement in housework and child care is likely to start for the sake of the mother's sanity and the continuation of the household, this involvement is also likely to have long-lasting and positive effects on the children.

High-Quality Baby Time: Fathers and Babies

"When I leave the house, I know I'm going to miss today's miracle," one father said. Martin Greenburg and Norman Morris did a study of fathers' reactions to their newborn babies, calling this new fascination "engrossment." New fathers would describe the infant as "perfect" and "beautiful." They wanted to keep touching the babies, holding them, looking at them. "I keep going back to him," said one father. "It's like a magnet."

Psychologists Lamb and Yogman have shown that babies learn to recognize their fathers very early. And they enjoy their fathers, because fathers tend to be more imaginative, unexpected, and physical in their play than women are. This seems to be an attribute of the maleness of fathers, not the fact they aren't home with the babies. Studies of fathers who are the primary caretakers of infants show that these men also handle the babies more vigorously and imaginatively than women tend to do.

Unfortunately, husbands whose wives go back to work early do not always have much opportunity to play with the baby. According to Lamb's studies, the two working parents compete for the limited amount of "alert, happy baby time" that is available in the evening. And the father often gets left out.

It is rather ironic, actually. The traditional idea was that if Mother stayed home with an infant and Father worked, Mother had some sort of "ownership" of the baby, and Father wasn't involved. Actually, by the end of the day, Mom would be eager to have a break from the baby, and Dad would be eager to play with him. When both parents work, the evening is often a parental competition for the limited "quality time" available. Mother is more likely to win this competition, and father's concern, engrossment, and investment in the child may have nowhere to go.

Some men might therefore choose to spend more evenings at work and less time at home. But as we will see in the next section, a father who is involved with his children can have a very important and very good influence on their development.

A Chip off the Old Block

Over and over, psychological studies and common sense come to the same conclusions about fathers: They can have a profound influence on how their children see the world and how well the children succeed in it. Sons of "involved" fathers (fathers who spend time with their boys) generally do better academically than the sons of less involved fathers. Fathers influence their daughters, also. Successful professional women often give credit to their fathers for inspiring them.

According to recent psychological research on fathering, the fathers that have the best effects on their children have several things in common:

- They are happy with their jobs. Men who feel powerless at work are more likely to be autocratic at home. Their children will try to avoid them rather than learn from them.
- They are kind. A father who is punishment oriented or who denigrates his children, frequently "loses" his children, who eventually turn out doing the same to *their* children.
- They are playful. One of the great things that a man can bring to the family is a sort of joyful and unexpected creativity.
- They share house work and child care. They are around for their children. Absent fathers or fathers who keep aloof from family life often have children with a variety of problems.

Some people worry, even in this enlightened age, that if a son sees his father doing housework and taking care of children, the son's sex-role identification will be seriously disturbed. Psychological research indicates that that is not the case. Henry Biller reviewed a great deal of work on the sex-role development of boys in the book *The Role of the Father in Child Development.* The main conclusion from Biller's work is that boys whose fathers are involved and kind and do some housework don't have any trouble knowing what the masculine role-model is. As a matter of fact, they follow the masculine model strongly, because they want to grow up to be like their fathers.

Nurturing the Mother: Shared Parenting

Within the past ten years, psychologists have "discovered" the role of the father in child development. Early research focused on how fathers played with infants, encouraged older children, were playful or punitive. In the last few years, however, researchers have noted other aspects of fathering: fathers interacting with mothers. The love between the parents is important to the child.

This common sense conclusion was supported by Frank Pedersen, of the National Institute of Child Health and Human Development. His pioneering study focused on how the father influences the family, rather than simply how he interacts with the baby. Pedersen concluded that fathers who were emotionally supportive of their wives usually had wives who were more effective mothers.

Pedersen noted that the emotional support that a man gives his child's mother begins in pregnancy. In the labor and delivery room, mothers who have loving husbands to support them tend to have easier labors. After the baby is born, the women who are emotionally supported by their husbands are more relaxed and effective with their babies. In the early days of parenting, the father nurtures the mother and the mother nurtures the child.

In order for the father to help the mother effectively, it is especially important that the two of them talk to each other about their expectations for child-care responsibilities. If the woman feels that because she's nursing he should do his part by changing all the diapers, and if he feels that he shouldn't touch diapers, there is going to be trouble. The real issue isn't even diapers, it is whether they can agree on responsibilities.

Luckily, communication is often easier for older parents. This was pointed out by several men we interviewed who had experienced fatherhood both early and then later in life. These men had fathered a child with their first wife while they were in their twenties. Now they were fathers for the second time, in their thirties or forties. One such father put it this way: "It was so much easier this time, mainly because we have some communication and coping skills. We have both had some practice in communicating under pressure."

But talking doesn't solve all problems. Communication alone will not ensure, for example, that the work is shared fifty-fifty. (See Chapter 8.) Neither husband nor wife should get too upset about this. Mothers get pregnant, fathers don't. Mothers give birth, fathers don't. Mothers lactate, fathers don't. During the pregnancy and the first year of the child's life, biology has very definite consequences. A child needs a loving mother and a loving father. It is not necessary that the two parents be interchangeable.

While the father will probably not involve himself in as much child care as the mother does, he still needs to be an active part of the family. Men often get a burst of job ambition after the baby is born, due to their increased responsibilities. Nevertheless, it is best if they hold this ambition in check for the first few months. You can't be supportive to your wife if you're not there.

Which brings up another question. All the other men at work are working such long hours. How is a man supposed to be supportive to his wife and still not lose his ability to support the family?

What About My Career? The Working Father

A father's involvement with the family can make a crucial difference to how relaxed and effective his wife is with the infant, to the older child's academic success, to his son's sex-role identification, to his daughter's career ambitions. What does that mean, however, on a day-to-day basis, for the real-life father? It's not as if he doesn't have a job. And some of his colleagues and competitors are fiends for hard work.

Of course the mother has similar problems. She has a job, and she too has colleagues, bosses, competitors. But the mother's and father's career philosophies often diverge for some time after the baby is born. The mother becomes aware that an extra hour at work is an hour away from the baby, and she begins to see her working life as a series of compromises. The father, on the other hand, often gets rededicated to his job. He doesn't want to just "play around," he wants to succeed and be a good provider. Especially now that his wife isn't working or working only part time, or else not as focused as she used to be.

In Chapter 9 we recommend that the mother take a few months' maternity leave, if possible. Should the father take paternity leave? Perhaps he should, but not many men do, not even in Sweden, where leave for fathers is protected by law. According to a recent article in the *San Francisco Chronicle,* one-fourth of the employers in Sweden said that they would "look less favorably" on a man who took paternity leave, even though such discrimination is illegal. Men just aren't expected to take paternity leave.

It would take a very strong willed man to go against society's expectations by asking for more than a few days of paternity leave. There are exceptions, of course. One self-employed man we interviewed took two months off when his first child was born. Another arranged for six weeks' leave without pay from his work. Both of them enjoyed their time off and were reluctant to return full time and leave the baby, but both felt pushed by economic necessity. The man who worked for an employer was also concerned with his employer's attitude toward his leave. Both were disappointed to discover that as soon as they went back to work they were doing far less than half of the baby care, a pattern that they and their wives had hoped to avoid.

Other men make arrangements to participate in child care on a more long-term basis. The new-mother accountant who quit the IRS (described in Chapter 3) works one day a week except during tax time. Her husband, a technical writer, works only four days a week. They share child care through the week, and only hire baby-sitters during the weeks before April 15.

How has this affected her husband's career? The good news is that he has received regular raises in the two years since the four-day-week arrangement started; nonetheless, he admits that he is very unlikely to get a promotion while working only four days. He is also unwilling to transfer to a different part of the company, for fear that other managers might not agree to continue his part-time program. In short, working four days a week has diminished his career options and changed his position from "regular guy, maybe the next manager" to "grateful that his manager will let him do this."

It happens that he doesn't want a promotion at this time; he is happy with the job he has. But if he ever wants to move up in the organization, he will have to work full time.

Of course, the same attitudes may well limit the options of a woman who takes extended leaves or who decides to work less than full time. A woman, however, may well inspire more corporate understanding. Her job might be affected, but people won't think her strange; it is considered natural for mothers to want to be with their children.

In short, very few men are likely to take any extended leave after the child is born or for child-rearing. How, then, can they be good fathers?

A GUIDE TO GOOD FATHERING: SHARED PARENTING

► Help the mother as much as possible when you are at home. Many new fathers do all the shopping and much of the housework. Baby care is also important: Mother needs a break for at least an hour each day. (See Chapter 8 for more on this.)

► For the first few months, the mother will probably be home and the father will be at work. This does not mean that they are not equal partners in the marriage; it does mean that during pregnancy and for the first year of a child's life, biological differences have practical consequences.

► Enjoy your baby's company in the evening. Babies get a lot out of playing with their fathers.

► Encourage the mother with praise and warm regard. Hopefully, in a good marriage, this will come easily. As one man said, "I think the sight of my wife nursing the baby was the most beautiful thing I've ever seen."

► You don't have to give up your job to be a good

father, but you can't work twelve hours a day, either. Babies can't bond with people they never see. Absent fathers can't help the mother very much. So don't quit, but work in moderation. After all, working fatherhood is a balancing act.

THE FATHER DEFINES HIMSELF: WHAT FATHERHOOD MEANS TO A MAN

Erik Erikson's landmark book, *Childhood and Society,* describes more than childhood. He also writes of the developmental tasks of adulthood. His ideas about these tasks have formed the basis for much psychological and popular literature on the subject, including Gail Sheehy's book *Passages.*

One of Erikson's adult tasks is "generativity," which he defines as "the concern in establishing and guiding the next generation"—in other words, for most men, the task of fatherhood.

Having a career is not a substitute for fatherhood. The career is a different life task than raising children is. (Erikson calls the career task "identity.") If a man opts out of involvement with his family, a marginally more successful career is not going to make up for what he missed.

Giving up on the family simply because your boss expects unlimited overtime is a good way for a man to cheat himself out of his own happiness, out of his own opportunities to achieve a fully adult life. It means letting someone else tell you what you need to do, rather than deciding for yourself. Ten years from now, when you have a different job, you may not remember much about your current boss' problems.

For a father in this society, the danger is in not achieving "generativity." There are many pressures to put your boss's need for your work above your family's need for your time.

But life tasks cannot be divided up this way. People in marriages can share work, but each person in a marriage has to achieve his or her own personal maturity. Which means that men need to have time for generativity, just as women get many opportunities for growth from their career time (identity).

Because, ultimately, parenthood is a profoundly important experience for adults of either sex.

Deciding

After sorting out the medical and financial issues, it seems that the choice should be simple, or at least manageable. The decision to have a baby is never the first important choice a woman of thirty has made. By the time she is thinking about having a baby, she has already decided about school courses, jobs, marriage. She has almost certainly bought a car or two and rented an apartment. She may have bought a house, gotten a divorce, gone back to school. Not all her decisions turned out to be perfect, but the process for making the choices seemed to work.

In contrast, the choice to be a mother seems so different, elusive, full of unknowns and ambivalence: "I can't imagine what's wrong with me. At the office I feel competent and in control, able to make decisions and give orders. But when I get home and relax, the baby question comes up again and my mind turns to mush."

After years of proving to yourself that you can manage your own life, why is this decision so difficult? No matter how intelligent and competent a woman is in other areas of her life, the same complaint invariably arises:

"Why can't I simply say yes or no and get on with my life?"

But the parenthood decision *is* different from all previous decisions. The choice to become a mother is the only major life decision that cannot be reversed. Husbands can be divorced and school can be re-entered after leaving it; people move to Majorca or Manhattan or sometimes back to their hometown. But being a parent is forever.

Because the choice is permanent, the thoughtful woman wants to do it "right." She sees her future with two branches. "I'm happy, now, with my decision not to have a child, but will I regret it when I'm sixty?" Or, "I really want a child, but I just don't know how I'll manage it."

The parenthood decision is life defining and permanent. If that weren't enough to frighten anybody, we must also mention that the results are entirely unpredictable. There is no way to know how you will feel about yourself, about your life as a parent, or even how your child might look or act at age one, five, ten, twenty. There is an element of risk, and the older we get the more risk-averse we often become. Living past our teenage years and early twenties makes us safer drivers but less daring decision-makers.

The purpose of this chapter is to help women make a decision about motherhood—help them get in touch with their own attitudes and hopes, organize their own sources of information, and review their medical and financial concerns. The exercises we present have helped hundreds of women, both in private counseling and at workshops all over the United States and Canada. But a decision about motherhood is rarely made in one day or on reading one chapter.

The motherhood decision is a process, a spiritual odyssey, not an event. It is an opportunity to confront dreams and fears, to discover new possibilities for commitment and personal growth. The process is not always orderly and progressive, but it does seem to go in steps, or stages, that are largely internal. Some exercises do help, and it is also worthwhile to know that seemingly irrational and troubled thoughts are part of the process, part of the experience of deciding.

Some women don't make an overt decision, yet still manage to decide. Younger women can delay: One woman, married at twenty-five, chose not to think about having children until she was at least thirty. Other women who are older and ambivalent about having children simply become less careful about birth control. The most extreme case of this method of deciding (at least, the most extreme case known to us) was a lawyer who stuck pinholes in her diaphragm but continued to use it. She had twins, a boy and a girl. Other women severely ambivalent about having a child keep saying "maybe" until their biological clock has definitely struck midnight. For them, "maybe" becomes a way of saying no, without confronting the potential problems of self-image that saying no implies.

But most women are uneasy with these partial solutions. For every woman who sticks a few pinholes into her diaphragm there are a hundred who want to decide carefully and firmly. They hope to time their pregnancies for health and for it to have a minimum effect on their working lives. For these women the question is, "How can I decide?"

The decision process may well take several months of self-searching. There are several steps to go through, and none can really be hurried. The first step is asking yourself the question, defining your dream by making a tentative choice. In the second step, you gather data, information, knowledge about the probable consequences of your choice. The third step is the most uncomfortable: We call it ambivalence and bargaining. This is the stage at which most women find the mental exercises in this chapter quite helpful. The next-to-the-last stage is integration; the choice becomes firmer, and much emotional energy goes into saying good-bye to the alternative. And the final stage is the decision: acknowledging it, acting on it, moving into the future you have chosen.

As you approach this watershed decision, you have your own set of concerns: your own health; relationship with husband or lover; career expectations; economic situation; memories of childhood; dreams and ideals of marriage, home, and family. The first step is recognizing where you are in the process.

STEP ONE: SELF-EVALUATION: CLARIFYING YOUR DREAM

Do you want to be a parent? Yes . . . No . . . Maybe. Now? Never? Later? A woman looks in her mirror one morning and realizes that this question has somehow shifted to the top of her "things to do today" agenda. For some women, a birthday triggers the question; for others, an unexpected illness causes thoughts of potential aging or physical vulnerability. Others link the parenthood choice-making process to a sense of achievement, not vulnerability. For them, a job promotion, a raise in salary, or buying a house is the trigger. The parenthood decision is made in a spirit of, "Well, we've finally gotten there, we're finally ready!"

Family expectations increase the pressure for some, possibly coming overtly from the grandparents-to-be. One woman remembers that her father-in-law would ask, "Do I hear a baby crying?" in a half-joking way, each time they spoke on the phone. Other family expectations are internal: "I suddenly noticed one day that my parents were growing old, my brother and my cousins all had children, and I was feeling left out of family celebrations. I had a dream of my family tree with me as a dead-end branch."

The trigger events can be subtle but powerful. For many women, the thirties are a decade of reevaluation of life goals at many levels, and age thirty-five marks a life shift. Gail Sheehy, in *Passages,* suggests that each life passage requires subtle changes in our perception of ourselves and a shift in our sense of aliveness or stagnation. "Is that all there is?" becomes the question to be answered. Or, as one woman put it, "Am I really getting somewhere with my life, or am I just commuting?" Some women are startled to find themselves looking into shop windows filled with baby clothes and suddenly noticing pregnant women.

Whatever the trigger event is, the process of reconsideration and clarification begins with deciding where you fit right now. Do you want to be a parent? Draw a grid, as Figure 1 indicates. Put an X (in pencil, not in indelible ink) in the box that describes your choice. If you have a husband or partner, place an O in the square to represent what you think his choice would be. The marks can always be erased later if you change your mind. But you have now set the stage by identifying the issue. Next comes exploring the terrain and writing the script.

	Yes	No	Maybe
Now			

	Yes	No	Maybe
Later			

Figure 1

STEP TWO: TESTING YOUR CHOICE AGAINST REALITY

Whatever box you checked in step one, the choice was tentative. At this stage, most women feel they need more information about the medical, psychological, financial, and social implications of their choice. This kind of reality testing may seem coldblooded when applied to such an emotional issue as having a baby. But most people who delay having a child do so for very practical reasons. It is time to consider:

- Health
  "I'm not sure I'm healthy enough." "I worry about having a healthy baby as I get older."
- Work and Economics
  "My job is so demanding." "I'm not sure I can work and be a good mother, too." "How can I support a child?"
- Relationships and Partners
  "I'm not sure that this marriage will last." "Can I really manage parenthood alone?"
- Personal Hopes and Fears
  "Is this really what I want to do?" "Do I want to be a mother for the rest of my life?"

Health

For women who have been careful about contraception for ten or twenty years and who have heard about the magic boundary-line of thirty-five, when one becomes an "elderly primagravida," the health questions are evident:

- How long can I wait to decide?
- What are the age-related medical risks for conception, pregnancy, and birth?
- How can I reduce the risks?
- How can I safely remain childfree, if I choose?

Chapter 2 contains guidelines for answering these questions. You might choose to learn more about your own health situation by scheduling a thorough checkup with your doctor at this time.

The last question, on remaining childfree, is not addressed at any length in this book. The major health consideration is safe, long-term contraception, since the pill, especially, is more risky for older women. Careful discussion with your gynecologist is important.

Work and Economics:

- The next major area of concern is work:
- How will my decision affect my work and career goals?
- How will I deal with the expenses of becoming a parent?
- How will I balance work and family responsibilities?
- What kind of mother do I expect to be, and how will this fit with my work situation?

Much of this book is devoted to guidance on these questions. Chapters 4 (financial planning for a baby), 8 (the first few months with the baby), 9 (the decision to go back to work), and 10 (choosing day care) are most relevant. This might also be the time to determine your own company's maternity leave policy, and assess your own income and fixed expenses.

A working woman is not the same as a working mother. Becoming a mother definitely adds a major role with additional demands on time, money, and energy. "I've thought about it a lot. My dream of happiness definitely includes a career and a family. I certainly intend to continue to work full time. I don't know just how it is going to be with a child, but I'm sure it will all work out." This is the typical situation: a goal but no strategy. Chapters 4 and 9 may help you formulate your own strategy.

Many women are concerned by the example other women set at work. Two women at Janet's company have had babies, and they both returned to work within a few weeks. "This is the kind of pressure I feel to prove I am equal to the men I work with. If I do have a baby and want to stay home for six months, what will happen to my job? Can I afford the risk?" We do not mean to minimize the pressure that Janet is under, but we do believe that every woman deserves to make her own decisions about her return to work. Ten years from now she may not even remember her former colleagues' names, but she will always remember whether or not she was comfortable with her decision.

The dual demands of work and motherhood can be overwhelming, and fear of these dual demands can cause some women to dismiss the idea of motherhood entirely. Occupations that welcome and honor maternity leaves are rare indeed. Every woman must explore her own options.

Once their baby is born, many women are surprised by their desire to stay home and fulfill the overwhelming needs of this new creature. A baby is not just an extracurricular activity. As one woman put it: "I knew it would be more work, when I had the baby. But I thought, What the heck, I managed night school. Let me tell you, having a baby is not at all like taking a couple of courses at night. I ended up extending my maternity leave for six months, after the fact. I really wish I had planned ahead better."

Part of planning ahead may be arranging for flexible hours for yourself. Some occupations lend themselves to at-home work or can be adapted to part-time hours. Free-lance copy-editing, computer programming from a terminal at home—these have worked for some people. Think about your own work, and if it can be adapted to part-time or stay-at-home work. Is your desire for a child strong enough to let you consider a temporary shift in work priorities?

This is also a good time to find out about day care. What is available, and how much does it cost? Chapters 9 and 10 provide some guidance on what to look for.

For the first year or two of a child's life, parenthood is not an equal-opportunity employer. Although husband and wife may both sincerely subscribe to a belief in fifty-fifty parenthood, the major responsibility for child care usually rests with the mother. Rare is the magazine article dealing with helpful hints for the working father! Planning for complementary rather than equal roles may be more realistic. Do you believe child care should be shared equally? Have you discussed these questions with your husband or partner? (More about this in Chapters 8 and 9.)

Which brings us from the area of work into the area of relationships.

Relationships and Partners

- What are my options for forming a family?
- How does my partner feel about fatherhood? Is he likely to be supportive and involved? Do we have the same expectations about parenthood and the same goals about style of living?
- How will my decision affect my relationships with friends and family?
- What is my support network like? Will I feel at ease as a parent, or will I feel isolated from my friends?

For many women, the fundamental reason for delaying parenthood is not having the ideal marriage or the ideal partner. As Linda described it, "Not having a baby was certainly not my dream. I always wanted to be a mother sometime, but only if I was married to a wonderful husband and father who would commit himself to fifty-fifty parenthood. I had been married in my twenties, but that didn't work out. When Prince Charming didn't ride into my life I considered having a child without marriage and bringing it up alone. I gave this a lot of thought, but decided that single parenthood wasn't for me. Now I really want to marry, and I'm looking for a potential father for the child I am ready for."

For some women, the ticking biological clock forces a shift from plan A (the ideal marriage) to plan B (the less-than-ideal marriage) to plan C (a willing partner) to plan D (no partner but the possibility of single motherhood), and on to plans E and F, which involve artificial insemination or adoption. As women get older, their options for achieving the ideal rose-covered cottage with a loving husband and 2.2 children begin to fade. If that is your position, Chapter 4 on the single mother provides a realistic assessment of what life may be like if you choose the parenthood option.

Even for married women, a husband may resist fatherhood. Sometimes he has children from a previous marriage and does not want more. More often, the current marriage is not "together" enough for both partners to agree on such a lifetime commitment. When this is the situation, having a baby is not a good solution for saving a marriage. See Chapter 8 for a description of the strains an infant poses to a relationship. Good marriages grow in this situation; shaky relationships are more often shattered.

Then there is the situation in which the man definitely wants a baby and the woman is less certain. Since the majority of baby care will probably rest on her shoulders for the first year (see Chapters 8, 9, and 10), having a baby must be a truly mutual decision. Although many marital conflicts can be resolved through compromise, there is no such thing as half a baby.

Personal Concerns

Besides relationships, there are internal goals; we all have our personal hopes, dreams, and fears. They are the source of our inner approval or disapproval for our actions:

- Why have I postponed the decision until now?
- What are my fantasies and fears about becoming a parent or remaining childless?
- What will I have to give up if I choose to be or not to be a parent? How can I be sure my decision will be right for me?

"I'll probably go on postponing the final decision. I think that having to come to terms with the decision is like coming to terms with the fact that you can't have it all in life. I feel that up to now in my life I've always been able to do what I wanted, and I've never been denied anything important. In this decision, I'm going to be denied something important one way or another—either my freedom and independence or the experience of being a mother. So I do feel torn. I spend a lot of time thinking about what it really means to have it all."

Trying to have it all may not be possible. Achieving

a lifelong high-pressure career, raising several children, having a perfect marriage, along with having friends, hobbies, leisure, exercise, health, peace of mind, happiness, and financial security seems to be volunteering for overload in one lifetime. But thinking in either/or terms is not necessary or helpful either. Women who are simultaneously involved in marriage, motherhood, and employment show the highest levels of well-being on many tests and the lowest levels of depression and illness. Of course, some people interpret this result another way: Only a very mentally healthy woman can consider working motherhood. (As they said about the pioneers on the Oregon Trail, "The cowards never started, and the weak died on the way.") It is more likely, however, that the roles of working woman and mother are complementary as often as they are contradictory, and the achievements in both spheres are a source of satisfaction.

There is no life that is free of stress, and a life without stress is neither possible nor desirable, because stress pushes us to action. A swimmer getting ready for a race is under stress, but he would not welcome the suggestion that he leave the pool, lie down on the couch, and take it easy. What a woman needs is not a stress-free life, but rather a pattern in which the rewards outweigh the problems. Being in the role you prefer is very important to well-being.

In terms of personal goals, the childbearing decision provides a unique opportunity to decide what rewards you really want to go after and what stresses you are willing to endure to get those rewards. There is no doubt that, at least for a few years, parenthood detracts from the energy available for a career. There is also no doubt that parenthood itself can be a tremendous experience of growth and maturation. *What do I want to accomplish with my life?* In many ways, it is the most exciting question anyone ever asked herself.

STEP THREE: AMBIVALENCE AND BARGAINING

Ambivalence is a state of uncertainty, and bargaining is the way we try to resolve the tension. It begins when, at some point, you will have collected enough information—read enough books, asked the experts, looked at and tried to answer the questions in step two—but the "right" answer is still elusive. "I feel as if I'm standing on a teeter-totter, perfectly balanced with one foot on each side, but I'm paralyzed. I can't move without giving something up." More simply: "Tell me what to do."

It is time to stop trying to think rationally about the choice and begin to trust your inner sense of knowing. Ambivalence is not emptiness. Groping through the confusion of uncertainty and doubt involves the work of the heart. It involves fantasizing, arguing with yourself, perhaps coming to terms with your attitudes toward your parents, toward parenthood, toward how you really feel about your partner, toward the extent of your ambitions for your career. It is not emptiness, but it isn't comfortable, either.

One exercise that has helped many women with this decision could be called "the phantom guarantee." If you could have three guarantees that would make you feel more comfortable with making a choice, what would they be?

Phantom Guarantees

1 _____

_____

_____

2 _____

_____

_____

3 _____

_____

Would they really tip the scales for you in one direction or another? If they would, are these guarantees actually possible in the real world? What equivalents are possible? Can you arrange those equivalents?

One woman wrote: "I would get pregnant right away if:

1 I could be absolutely sure I would have a healthy baby.

2 I could take a nine-month leave from my job and then work part-time.

3 I could find excellent, cheap child care for my baby."

Probably a common dream, and not one with much probability of coming true *as it is stated.* Holding on to these exact expectations could keep this woman from ever taking a chance on motherhood. But if she did enough information gathering and reality testing, she would be able to look at these guarantees again, in a real-world sense.

1 Is there a reason that she has a much greater-than-average chance of bearing a child with a serious birth defect or hereditary disease? If not, is she still too uncomfortable to take the average chance with pregnancy?

2 How long a leave can she take from work? What are the financial constraints? The job constraints? How does she feel about these possibilities?

3 What kind of child care would she be comfortable with? How much can she afford to spend? Does she have relatives who might help out part time? Can she and her husband arrange flexible schedules to share some child care?

Another woman wrote: "I really don't want to be a mother, but:

1 I never want to regret my choice.

2 I don't want to be criticized for being selfish.

3 I don't want to miss something important."

Again, a set of dreams and guarantees pretty much unrealizable. But there may be real-world equivalents that will make this woman more comfortable with her choice to remain childless. For example, "I don't want to be criticized for being selfish." It would be impossible to arrange that nobody in the world will ever accuse a given childless woman of being selfish. Rude people are everywhere. But this woman was probably not talking about the opinions of strangers at parties. Perhaps she really means "I don't want my mother to call me selfish." If she can restate the problem this way, she may be able to deal in an effective and adult way with her relationship with her mother. What if her mother does call her selfish? What does she think her reaction will be? What should her reaction be?

No matter what imaginary or real guarantees you are hoping for, it is important to recognize and trust your own decision-making style. Will you be reassured if you do a careful financial analysis, or would you think more clearly taking a hike up a mountain?

It is time to trust yourself. There are many paths to understanding what your heart wants to do. You will know whether yes or no is your answer. Or you may still be uncertain. Perhaps you need to go back to an earlier step in the process: Is there some information about finances or birth defects that you feel you need to have? Is there some concern with a significant relationship that you need to really face?

STEP FOUR: INTEGRATION, FANTASY, AND LETTING GO

When a decision is being made internally and the scale is tipping, we begin to mentally rehearse, "What it would be like if. . . ." We also begin to say good-bye to the road not taken. Genuine transitions depend upon leaving something behind. The root of the word *decide* is in the Latin "to cut off," the cutting off of other choices. Cutting off involves a mourning process, giving up something, nostalgia and sorrow for the path that will never be explored. Nobody has it all, no matter what decision is made. Fantasy, considering the road not taken and the road to be taken, are important parts of this decision stage.

One exercise that has helped many women rehearse and solidify their decisions involves something that might be called the "life-map." In some ways, it presents a variation on the "What do you want to have written on your tombstone?" question that is often used to help people define their goals. But the life-map is a little more cheerful; it involves fantasizing about life.

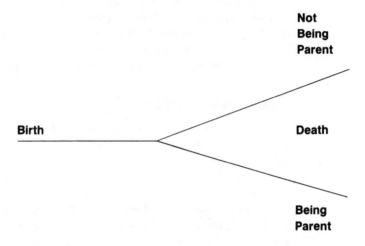

Figure 2

Use a large sheet of paper and some colored crayons or felt pens. Following the format in Figure 2, draw your life. Identify your birth on the left side, your present age as a point somewhere in the middle. Write the word *death* on the far right side. Fill in the important people, events, and turning points from your birth until now with words or symbols. From the point representing your current age, divide the paper into two sections, one labeled "parent" and the other, "nonparent." Fill in these two sections with words and symbols describing your fantasy of that choice in your life. Do this alone. Then ask your partner to do it also. Compare and talk with each other about your life-maps. Take plenty of time to do this. Our inner thoughts need encouragement and quiet space to emerge. Not everyone feels comfortable using this technique, but for those who use it, it has made a real difference. It helps you see yourself as someone who has decided. The life-map will clarify and solidify your decision. But you may find it reassuring or unsettling to see what you think and hope life holds.

Your life-map will be a unique creation, but to show you what others have done, Figure 3 presents a life-map drawn by one woman facing the parenthood decision. Yours may of course have more or less detail, depending on the considerations you need to work through.

STEP FIVE: DECISION AND ACTION

A decision is tentative until it is honored by action. At this stage, if you still feel a strong inner resistance to the decision, it may be necessary to go back to an earlier step of the process and try to look at the problem and resolve it. Perhaps do the "phantom guarantee" exercise again.

Usually, however, there is no such major problem . . . just an uneasiness. How to be sure that you are sure, *really sure*. Well, there is no such thing as *really sure*. The car you didn't buy isn't unattractive just because you chose differently. There was a virtue to that other car, or you wouldn't have looked at it. Of course, it is easier to accept that you can't buy every car on the market than it is to accept that you can't have it all in your life. But both are really acceptances of the limits of what one person can do.

Assume, for a moment, that your decision is parenthood. An agenda for action may help at this stage. Draw a large circle and divide it into four sections representing your priorities for action about health, work, relationships, and personal issues. Each of these four will receive a proportionate share of your 360 degrees of action energy. Then, for each of these four, list what you want or need to do in order to begin to make things happen. Perhaps

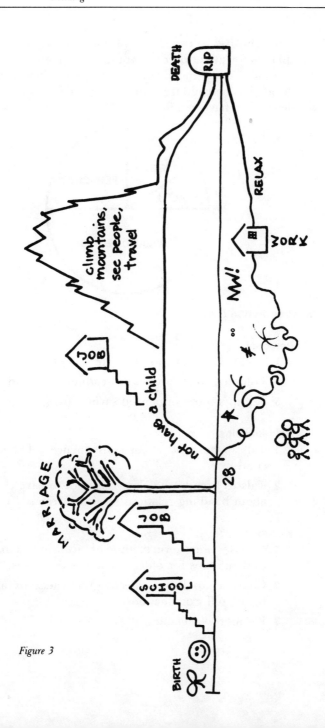

Figure 3

you want to take care of health now and leave the other spheres for attention once you get pregnant.

Here are two action plans, one made by a woman who decided to be child free, and one made by a woman who decided to have a child.

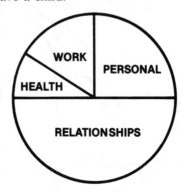

Childfree Action Plan

Personal

1 Decide on return to graduate school.

2 Volunteer once a week to read for the blind.

3 Set up a more organized savings plan.

Relationships

1 Talk to husband about consequences of remaining child free.

2 Talk to friend, who also chose not to have children, about handling relationship with parents.

Health

1 Choose a long-term method of birth control that isn't as dangerous for older women as the pill is.

2 Continue to have gynecological checkups and do breast self-examinations.

3 Eat more vegetables.

Work

1 Ask for more challenging assignments.

2 Arrange to go on more business trips.

3 Join the Toastmasters International public-speaking club.

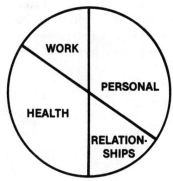

Parenthood Action Plan

Personal

1 Make an agenda for pre-baby self-indulgences.

2 Spend time with myself.

3 Buy some good books on parenting.

Relationships

1 Talk to husband about fatherhood.

2 Talk to friends who are parents.

3 Ask friend if we can occasionally swap baby-sitting.

Health

1 See physician.

2 Stop smoking.

3 Find out about prenatal exercise classes.

4 Gain five pounds.

5 Eat more vegetables.

Work

1 Check health insurance maternity benefits.

2 Find out options for time out from work.

3 Review overall economic status.

Are you ready now to make out your own agenda? If not, perhaps you need to go back to some of the earlier exercises. Or perhaps reading the second half of this book, about pregnancy, birth, and life with a baby, can help you decide.

Pregnancy and Beyond

One Baby, a Thousand Miracles: The Pregnancy Experience

Pregnancy is an active situation, not simply a period of passive waiting. The pregnant woman goes through intense physical and emotional changes. She reevaluates her career, is concerned with her changing body image, rethinks her relationship with own mother, dreams about her own motherhood role. Then there's the man responsible for the pregnancy: Carrying his child changes that relationship. There are new needs for a different type of female friendship, supportive colleagues of motherhood.

This mixed bag of miracles may seem overwhelming when it appears as a list, yet every one of us is the result of a successful pregnancy. How do women make the adjustments? It depends on the woman.

Fortunately, the older and mature woman usually has an easier time dealing with these concerns and reevaluations. As we noted in our discussion of the effect of maternal age on child-rearing, readiness and maturity still count. The older woman is more likely to be at ease with herself, as a competent person and as a woman.

For all women, pregnancy is incontrovertible proof of

womanhood and of sexual activity. As such, it can be profoundly embarrassing to a woman who is working in a man's profession. She may not even really know why she is embarrassed. One attorney burst into tears when she told her boss she was pregnant. She felt she had let him down. A female police officer spent an inordinate amount of time worrying about whether the gun belt was going to fit around her expanded waistline. She was also concerned with an indefinable "loss of authority" while pregnant. There is no doubt about it: Once you are pregnant, it is hard to be one of the boys.

This chapter is a guide to the many changes and reassessments that come with pregnancy. The first section describes the physical and emotional changes of pregnancy on a trimester-by-trimester basis; the second describes some predictable emotional issues, such as changes in the relationship to the baby's father. We do not, however, include one very important topic: physical preparation for childbirth. This was a deliberate omission. The shelves are full of excellent and comprehensive books on preparation for labor and delivery (recommended reading on childbirth is listed in the reference section at the back of the book). Also, older mothers often take a childbirth education class, which inundates them with literature, charts, and illustrations.

How childbirth is managed is very important, of course. But, after all, labor and delivery usually take less than twenty-four hours. In other countries, these hours are shrouded in mystery; in America, they are the subject of much study and conversation. There is no doubt that a woman who informs herself, carefully prepares for childbirth, gets good medical care, and is unanesthetized during labor is doing what is best for the baby. But motherhood is not determined in that one fateful day. Preparation for motherhood does not just mean preparation for childbirth. The emotional work of pregnancy is also vital, to prepare for the changes the baby will bring in your life.

SYMPTOMS OF CHANGE: THE TRIMESTER TALLY SHEET

As a woman goes through pregnancy, her perception of the reality of the baby changes. During the first trimester, she adjusts to the fact that she is really pregnant. The second trimester, she reassures herself that there is actually something in there, something that kicks, that has a heartbeat. And the third trimester, she once again faces the fears she faced in the first trimester. What is childbirth going to be like? Will the baby be all right?

First Trimester: The First Twelve Weeks

At first, pregnancy feels like a mild stomach upset. The odors of cooking seem unbearably strong, and testiness and irritability are common. Marjorie Karmel, the author of *Thank You, Dr. Lamaze,* describes early pregnancy in Paris. "Suddenly I began to feel nervous and upset. I gave up wine for a few days. In France wine can explain a lot of things. But I continued to feel peculiar. I even began to consider going to a doctor. Then suddenly I was struck by an idea. I sat down with a calendar. . . ." Another symptom is the feeling that your period is just about to start—a bloated, heavy-breasted feeling. But menstruation doesn't begin.

These feelings are caused by the immense hormonal changes going on in your system. Progesterone is relaxing the muscles that form the wall of the blood vessels, causing circulatory changes that can leave the mother dizzy or light-headed. The same hormone is slowing down the gastrointestinal tract, causing digestive upsets and nausea.

It seems clear that the extent of a woman's symptoms at this stage will be determined by the exact mix of hormones in her blood, her body's response to this, her attitude, and her environment. Attitude can be significant, but the whole business of the importance of attitude in early pregnancy is usually carried too far. One book claimed that women who were not at all nauseated during the first few months were "denying" their pregnancy. On the other hand, women who were vomiting a great deal were "rejecting" their pregnancy. According to these (male) psychologists, there is a correct and appropriate degree of nausea that should be caused by progesterone's effect on the gastrointestinal tract. And these men feel that the degree of discomfort is a clear indication of the woman's mental health.

Nonsense! Early pregnancy is a time of great stress on the mother's body. All sorts of systems must be put into place to nurture the embryo. Hormonal levels change rapidly, and the rest of the body sort of tags along behind, adjusting as best it can. The physical problems of the first trimester are seldom serious, and most women, most of the time, will take the symptoms in stride. This is not the same as saying that the whole thing is psychosomatic, or an attention-getting device, or rejection, or denial.

Along with the physical discomfort, the first three months can bring on a period of intense ambivalence about having a baby, which is often coupled with a fear of miscarriage. Husbands sometimes find their wives absolutely incomprehensible in these early months: "Do you want the baby or don't you? What's the *matter?*" The matter is that the woman is dealing with hormonal and body changes that are beyond her control and not very pleasant. She also needs more sleep, but she is probably continuing to work full time at her job. Her digestive system is out of kilter, and her breasts feel swollen and tender.

Most of all, she is beginning to be aware of the commitment she has made. She is pregnant. She's not thinking about being pregnant. She's no longer weighing her options. She's made her choice, and the only way out of this situation is through giving birth. And this ambivalence describes the woman who wanted to get pregnant! The woman who wasn't sure she wanted to get pregnant may feel worse; for her, the physical and emotional adjustments can be overwhelming.

But hang on. The second trimester (months three through six) is coming.

The Second Trimester: The Thirteenth to Twenty-sixth Week

In the second trimester, all systems are in place for the baby. Your body has adjusted to the hormone levels, and there is little or no nausea. Early milk (colostrum) may leak from your breasts. You feel the first gentle kicks from within. This evidence convinces you that you are really pregnant—not sick, but actually carrying a child. Your skin may be rosy in color (probably from increased blood supply), and people may compliment you on how well you look. This is the madonna phase, when most women are comfortable, even a bit smug. The concern now is weight gain. For the first trimester, you wore your regular clothes, but now there's no doubt about it—you look "fat," you feel heavy. It's time for the maternity clothes. But it is time also for hearing the baby's heartbeat through the doctor's stethoscope, for feeling those little kicks, and for dreaming.

The second trimester has its darker side for older mothers. This is when amniocentesis, described in Chapter 1, to determine the genetic makeup and possible birth defects of the child, is administered.

"I don't know why they talk about the trimesters of pregnancy," one woman said. "Pregnancy has three stages: before the amniocentesis, waiting for the results, and after the results." For many older mothers, this is very true. Everything is put on hold for twenty weeks, until the results are available and the healthiness of the child is confirmed.

In most cases, everything is fine. One woman calculated that she had run a 0.5-percent chance of miscarriage from the amnio procedure in order to diagnose a 1-percent chance of a Down's syndrome child. "I wouldn't do it again," she said. "Not for a 0.5-percent gain." (This was comparatively easy for her to say, after having had two healthy children.)

For other people, a negative amniocentesis result can mean a painful time of decision. "I began to scream as soon as I heard [the doctor's] voice. . . . I knew that only [negative] results are reported by phone [rather than by mailing a card]. The image of myself, alone, screaming into the white plastic telephone is indelible." Thus Rayna Rapp described, in *Ms.* magazine, her reaction to the news that she was carrying a Down's syndrome child.

Rapp went ahead and had a late abortion. A late abortion is very different from an early abortion. After a late abortion, the woman's body reacts as if there had been a birth. The breasts fill with milk, which adds to the physical and emotional pain. As Rapp describes it, "I had no idea that deep mourning for a fetus could be so disorienting."

Nevertheless, she did not wish to raise an afflicted and severely handicapped child. The majority of women who learn they are carrying a Down's syndrome child make the same decision. Hopefully, in the future, the decision can be made earlier, through chorionic villi sampling, which is now being tested, as described in Chapter 2. Any necessary abortions could then take place in the first trimester, when the fetus is at a much earlier stage of development and the mother's commitment to the pregnancy is less developed.

It should be noted, however, that the incidence of Down's syndrome, though increasing with age, is only 1 percent at age 35 and 2 percent at age forty (these are the most negative figures we have available; see Chapter 2 for other estimates). For most older mothers, the comfortable second trimester is made even happier, because it is the trimester when they hear the *good* news.

The Third Trimester: The Twenty-seventh to Thirty-eighth Week

The third trimester (months seven through nine) is more difficult. At this point, the baby is gaining weight at a rate of half a pound a week, and the mother may be gaining even faster. A surprising number of mothers use the term "beached whale" to describe themselves during this time. It describes both how they imagine they look and how they feel: a fish out of water, awkward, motionless. The baby's kicks are no longer gentle. When the baby shifts positions, the mother's entire abdomen moves from side to side. One woman relates that she felt like a canary cage with a buffalo inside.

Depression may come—the feeling that things are out of control, fear of stretch marks, of becoming permanently fat, not being young anymore. Increased dependence on your husband (or others) is common. There is often severe impatience with the pregnancy.

In some ways, the third and first trimesters are rather similar. There is physical discomfort both times—nausea the first trimester, bulkiness and disturbed sleep in the last trimester. There is concern with how the baby will change your life, whether delivery will be painful, whether the baby will be all right. Vivid and troubling dreams are common now, in which the baby may be deformed, or else is all right but dies of neglect. These dreams are part of the anxiety-preparation for motherhood.

And once again, as in the first trimester, is the realization that the only way out of this situation is childbirth.

CONTROL AND SURRENDER: THE BIRTH PROCESS

Birth is the climax, the transition, the end of pregnancy— and the beginning of motherhood.

Labor is an unpredictable experience for women of every age. Labor starts when it is going to start, and not on any schedule. The last weeks of pregnancy are often filled with minor false alarms, preliminary contractions signaling that the uterus is getting ready for a birth. Each time, the woman wonders: Will the contractions get stronger, should I tell someone, go to the hospital? Is this it? Usually, the contractions get weaker; they fade away. The suspense can be maddening. The dominant emotion of the last two or three weeks of pregnancy is impatience.

For a first-time mother, another feeling is fear. What will labor be like? Will the baby be healthy? The older mother, especially, is ready to blame any deviation from perfection on herself. She shouldn't have waited; that's the reason for everything. As discussed in Chapter 2, very few birth problems are actually associated with age (see Table 1 in that chapter, especially). The same is true of length of labor.

What is labor like? It is labor, hard work. One older mother said, "You know, when I saw the childbirth movie, I guess I thought that the woman grunting and getting red in the face was doing that for effect, to get sympathy. I just couldn't believe that my body could work that hard. In my own labor, I had to bear down a long time to push the baby out. It just seemed to take forever. Muscles in my arms were quivering uncontrollably from gripping those hand-hold things to anchor myself while I pushed. I said to my husband, 'I can't believe how hard it is.' Not so much pain as hard work."

There is pain, too. A prepared mother who knows how to react can handle the pain. It is, after all, intermittent. There is usually a rest between the contractions, except for a brief period (the transition) just before the cervix opens fully. For an unprepared mother, or for a mother who believes her preparation should put her into a sensationless nirvana, the contractions can be overwhelming. It is not so much that the pain is so bad, but that it is a symptom of the uterus taking over. The uterus is getting that baby out, and the mother is just along for the ride, like it or not.

A prepared labor implies a labor coach. During the birth itself, the labor coach's encouragement and support (and perhaps even his or her coaching) can give the mother reassurance that she is doing well and that she is not alone. Studies have shown that mothers who have labor coaches also tend to have shorter and easier labors and are more relaxed with the brand-new baby.

But "shorter" and "easier" are relative terms. Labor is still labor. Having a baby is a profoundly shocking experience. Nothing in a modern woman's life prepares her, really, for the immense effort involved. Perhaps marathon runners are prepared. They run through exhaustion, through "hitting the wall." They may be partially prepared.

For ordinary women, who don't run marathons, the best preparation is to know what is happening, to know what parts of the event are within your control (breathing, pushing) and what parts are outside your control (length of labor, condition of the baby). It is an experience unparalleled in its intensity, something that is nothing like whatever has happened before in your life.

There can be ecstasy, also. Nothing in the world can possibly be as satisfying as the moment the baby emerges and starts crying lustily. Every nerve fiber in the mother's body rejoices with that glad cry. The sense of accomplishment and relief are amazing. One woman said, "Now I know the meaning of the word euphoria. I didn't know before. I thought it just meant happiness."

In short, words cannot express the physical stress and the spiritual joy of childbirth; but words can express some of the psychological pitfalls. For the older mother, the major problem is an exaggerated opinion of how much of the process she can expect to control. This opinion can easily lead to an unrealistic sense of disappointment that she didn't do well enough. When unrealistic expectations on the part of the mother (to do it all herself, perfectly) are coupled with conservative treatment on the part of the doctor, the chances for disappointment are many. Some women feel they have failed if the doctor uses medical procedures (forceps, anesthesia) during an unpredictably difficult labor. A well-prepared mother must still be psychologically flexible enough to appreciate that there may be a need for medical intervention.

Birth is the first experience of parenting. It may be the first time that you realize that all you can do is your best —but that you really can't take full responsibility for the outcome. In that sense, matching expectations with reality in birth, as well as forgiving yourself for any deviation from your ideal, is good practice for the years to come.

You do your best with the birth, and move on to the next challenge: bonding with the baby.

INSTANT BONDING: NECESSARY OR NONSENSICAL?

As recently as ten years ago, babies were snatched from the delivery room by the hospital staff and not returned to the mothers until hours later. There was no chance for the mother to hold and admire her baby. After a normal birth, babies are often in a quiet, alert state for about an hour. That first hour is an excellent time for mother and baby to get to know each other. Hustling the baby away was an extremely unkind thing to do. A mother who wants to touch her baby but is left with empty arms is more prone to depression.

Recently, however, the hospital pendulum has swung to a new extreme. There's a strong feeling that the first hour of "imprinting" is crucial. After giving birth, women are supposed to be taking part in the biological mystery of bonding. Many women are terribly afraid that they are not doing it right. If the woman has had a cesarean, she's busy having abdominal surgery during that "crucial" bonding time. If there was a difficult delivery, mother and baby may fall asleep. Has the chance for bonding passed? If you don't do it in the first hour, are you ever going to do it?

One woman said, "When I had the cesarean, I felt so bad about it. I knew I should be bonding with him, but I wasn't able to. For the first six weeks, every time he cried and wouldn't be comforted, I wondered if it was because of the bonding I missed."

Susan Goldberg reviewed the literature on parent-infant bonding in an article in *Child Development* magazine. She concluded that early studies of the effects of delivery-room contact on mother-infant bonding were seriously flawed. In the original data, no study really showed a long-lasting effect of delivery-room contact between mother and infant. There seemed to be short-term beneficial effects or else no effects on later relationships.

However, the studies did indicate that the presence of a supportive companion for the mother during labor was of great importance. "Women who had a supportive companion during labor and delivery did more talking, stroking, and smiling in their first contacts with their infants than those who labored alone. . . . The presence of a supportive companion was also associated with a shorter labor, fewer delivery complications, and more time awake for the mothers during their . . . interaction period with the infant." In short, women who have support during labor have an easier time of the birth and more energy and love to give to the infant postpartum.

A word about bonding and fathers: Like mothers, fathers who have prepared for childbirth with their wives are often prepared to be coaches for delivery but not prepared for the reality of fatherhood. As one father said, "After the birth, the doctor asked me to hold the baby and give her to my wife. Then he asked me to help weigh the baby. I was terrified. It was an intensely emotional experience for me, holding her like that. I got used to her, a little bit, while they were still working with my wife. It was amazing. They had never told me anything about the baby when we were getting ready for the birth."

This experience may actually have a longer-term effect. According to Goldberg's article, father-infant contact in the delivery room has a definite, positive effect on how involved the father is with the infant later. The effect is better documented than early bonding effects of the mother-infant pair.

One possible explanation of this phenomenon is that mothers will interact with and bond with their infants no matter what happens in the delivery room. But fathers can be rather shy of a newborn. When the father is invited to hold the child immediately, when the doctor confirms the father's role as part of the team, part of the family, then the man's initial shyness ("I was terrified") can be quickly overcome.

To summarize the latest research on "bonding" right after birth: Anything that supports the family as a family (support for the mother in labor, involvement of the father with the infant) is likely to help the human process of bonding. Overall, human bonding is a process that starts with birth, not an event that takes place on the delivery table. But remember, there are some excellent mothers who have said, "I don't think I really loved her until she was a couple of weeks old." There is plenty of time, after delivery, to get to know and love your baby.

But before we go on (in Chapter 8) to describe the further work of learning to be a mother, we should finish discussing some other issues that arise during pregnancy.

EMOTIONS IN MOTION: PREDICTABLE ISSUES OF PREGNANCY

"Do you think of yourself as a mother yet?"

"Not at the moment. I've spent almost twenty years of my life avoiding motherhood. I feel as if it will take another twenty to revise my thinking."

All over the world, there is some celebration when a woman bears her first child. With this event, the new mother takes on an enhanced status. For the over-thirty working woman, however, the status shift is unclear and complex. "I felt I was taking on a great burden for myself. I felt I needed to apologize a lot for being pregnant."

Only part of the adjustment is learning to think of yourself as a mother. The most difficult adjustment seems to be in facing multiple, constantly shifting issues. "I just get one thing settled, and then another comes up."

Although each pregnancy is unique, there are some universals. For one thing, pregnant women are often emotional. Highs and lows come and go swiftly. Of course, many women take pains not to show this, especially if they are in an office environment. But reading in the newspaper about the death of a child may bring a shower of tears. At other times a woman may feel wonderfully special, like a child with new shoes, a new dress, and an ongoing birthday party. She may want to sing, just walking down the street.

Such emotionalism is actually necessary, no matter how inconvenient. It would be impossible for a woman to work through so many life adjustments in nine months without being in touch with her emotions. So nature and hormones arrange for her feelings to be closer to the surface, even if she begins to worry that she's never going to be logical again.

The most outward change is her expanding body, filled with a growing baby. But the changes in her own psyche are just as profound and mysterious. Ready or not, she faces reevaluation of

- her body image and sense of control
- her changing roles and relationships
- child care and mothering expectations
- career commitment and friendships
- sexual relationship with her partner.

Body Image and Sense of Control

The first issue is body image. In other centuries and in other places, the pregnant body has approached the ideal. Nowadays, the marathon runner has the ideal shape. Many women spend most of their lives on diets to lose or control weight. This makes the shape-changes of pregnancy hard to accept. Not only do you declare to all the world that you are a woman, but you become a "fat" woman simultaneously.

Most women adjust to these changes. Some may over-eat, in order to "grow the baby," do something for it. These women are delighted when they start to "show." Others carefully read the scale, and get distressed if they are gaining more than they "should." These women console themselves that soon pregnancy will be over, at which time they'll get back to their svelte, prepregnant state. As one woman said, "I tell myself that Raquel Welch had a kid. She must have been fat and pregnant once!"

How does the woman feel about the loss of control that goes with her expanding body? The more distressed she is about loss of control, the more disturbed she will be at her heavy breasts and swollen abdomen. If her husband is also obviously distressed by her appearance, if he mocks her, then her problems with self-image will be worse.

There may be an added fear: "I'm ugly, will he leave me now?" On the other hand, many men find the pregnant body very sexy. It helps if one of these men is the husband, and he's not afraid to express himself.

For single women, the growing body must be explained somehow. There must be a prepared line, something to say. One woman commented, "Everybody said the same thing: 'You're pregnant; I didn't even know you were married!' Then I'd say, 'I'm not married.' Then they would stand there, apologizing and tripping over themselves. So I began saying, "I'm not married; I always wanted to be a mother, not a wife.' Actually, it's a lot more complicated than that, but I had to say something."

For all women, attendance at a prenatal/postpartum exercise class can help you adjust to your new body. By seeing other women in various stages of their heaviness, you can affirm the correctness, appropriateness, and beauty of your own new shape.

Changing Roles and Relationships: The Father and Others

Father/Husband

Pregnancy is also the beginning of the adjustment of the couple to their new roles as parents. This adjustment between husband and wife is often difficult. The man may be turned off by her pregnant body; he may be mystified by her mood swings. He may also feel excluded. His wife's attention turns inward, away from him. Some men are actively jealous of the baby. This is an awkward situation, especially since many men often cannot acknowledge such negative feelings, even to themselves. At the same time, he may be delighted and proud, if parenthood was something he really desired.

The concerns above apply to any father of any age. But older couples have some special problems. They usually have an unspoken marriage contract, which has been operative for a long time. The contract usually involves the wife working, and the husband and wife sharing financial responsibility and household arrangements. Frequently, the woman has made a minor domestic art of planning things that will keep her man happy—arranging for concert tickets, making his favorite dinner, planning ski trips with friends. In some ways, he is like her "only child." Suddenly, all of this is jeopardized.

The woman is obsessed with her pregnancy. She's not sure when she will go back to work or how much infant day care will cost. She is thinking about her husband in a new way: What will he be like as a father? Their financial arrangements, her concern with his comfort, her self-sufficiency—everything is changed. The marriage obviously needs a new contract, one in which the wife is allowed to be more dependent on the husband, through his increased emotional support. Such new contracts are seldom easy.

Childbirth education classes that both husband and wife attend can help with this transition. The husband as coach is a role that both partners can enjoy as they make the necessary adaptations. One man bought himself a set of T-shirts with COACH on them, which he wore around the house. Another woman, very independent before pregnancy, told her friend, "The Lamaze classes are just like obedience school, and I'm the puppy!" The classes provide a safe zone, a mutual involvement in the pregnancy, which can help the couple work out their other adjustments.

Daughter, Mother, Grandmother

While most pregnant women have a husband, every pregnant woman had a mother. The mother-daughter relationship is key to a woman's understanding of her own identity. This relationship becomes reconsidered. "So this is what she went through to have me." The new mother may be afraid of not measuring up to the standards of her own mother, or she may fear being as insufficient a mother, being all the things she doesn't want to be. There may be irrational fears that the new grandmother will "steal" the baby. This may be coupled with the more rational fear that the grandmother will "take over" if she comes to visit after the birth. A woman makes her child-care decisions in the context of her own experience with her own mother.

If a woman's relationship with her own mother is uncomfortable, the intense identification with the mother that comes with pregnancy may not be very pleasant. Nevertheless, working through these feelings is what the psychologists call an "important developmental task." A woman who is about to become a mother must consider, at both rational and irrational levels, how her own mother took care of her. What was wrong, what was right? How does she want to take care of her own baby?

This reconsideration can be especially difficult for the older mother, who has been certain that she has defined her life fairly completely. A woman past thirty usually believes that she has been making her decisions free of concerns about what her mother would want her to do. It can be extremely upsetting when the old conflicts and the old uncertainties surface again. Suddenly, she realizes that there is an entire aspect of her life that she has not yet handled: She has not yet given birth to or cared for a baby.

At one level, the mother-to-be may be more forgiving and more in touch with her own mother. At another level, her hard-won sense of differentiation (she does things this way, but I do things that way) may be undergoing siege. Again, this crisis is a bit harder for the average older mother, who has had longer to think that the question of "who I am" has been resolved.

There is no simple formula for working this matter through. Careful thought about child-rearing can be valuable in resolving the conflicts. Talk to other women who are contemporaries of yours about their child-care decisions, their relationships with their mothers. Gather together a group of friends who will support you in your own decisions.

In other cases, the grandmother will actually be in charge of the child while the mother goes back to work. This used to be quite common, especially among immigrants. Even today, such arrangements are more common than the newspapers, with their focus on large day-care centers, would have you believe. Of course, in this case, the grandmother's approach to child care must be compatible with how the mother wants things done, or else the stage will be set for real trouble.

Child Care and Mothering Expectations

Whether a grandmother is available or not, thinking about baby care is an obvious part of the work of pregnancy. Surprisingly, however, this issue usually doesn't weigh much on a woman's mind until fairly late in the pregnancy, frequently not until the last month. This may be short-sighted, but then there's a lot of other emotional work to do, before the actual baby can be considered. It is common for women to have "panic attacks" about lifestyle changes in the last month of pregnancy.

Sometime in the third trimester the reality of the baby is acknowledged. This is the time for buying the crib, the layette, the book on breastfeeding, for selecting a pair of names. This is another instance where exercise classes come in handy. Watching other women make the transition to motherhood can be very reassuring.

Career Commitment and Friendships

One area that may waver in focus during pregnancy is that of job commitment. With all the feelings you need to work through about your body, your mother, your husband, and your baby, it is not very surprising that there is little energy left over for your normal office work load, much less office politics.

The job, however, is a fact of life. Few older women choose to quit forever as soon as they hear the good news. Instead, they turn their job-related energies to topics of interest to them: arranging maternity leave, negotiating for part-time work for a few months after the baby comes, finishing up important projects. Chapter 3, on financial planning for the baby, has practical suggestions for this period.

Despite the time constraints, there is something one should take care to initiate and maintain: friendship with other mothers. Mothers in the "women's quarters" of Arabic societies have support, good advice, and friendship near at hand, as well as rivalries. Primitive women are assisted by older and wiser midwives. Only in the Western world are women so isolated.

Friendship with other mothers can be very important. Phyllis Chesler, author of *Women and Madness,* describes a conversation with a famous older mother in her pregnancy journal, *With Child:*

"Margaret Mead paid me a visit today. . . . She insisted on coming to see me, because 'being pregnant is more fragile a state than being old.' As she comes in, removing her cape, positioning her walking stick, her question, before we sit down, is: 'What are you doing about your nipples?' This is something my own mother hasn't asked. I say, 'Nothing.'

'Rub them with a rough washcloth, pinch them, toughen them up,' she tells me. Bluntly. Simply. . . .

"We talk about the problems that arise when a 'professional' woman becomes pregnant 'late in life.' As she did at thirty-eight. As I'm doing at thirty-seven. 'What happens is significant and incredibly joyful,' she assures me, 'If you have your work and enough money.' "

How reassuring that conversation was for the expectant mother! It had practical advice on how to prepare for breastfeeding, and hopeful discussion of life after the baby. But the same reassurances, perhaps without the same weight of authority, could be received by any woman from friends who are mothers. Of course, there is always the possibility of bad advice, but the discussion would still be valuable. Isolation is always worse than occasional bad advice.

Sex and Pregnancy: A Nine-Month Guide to a Personal Issue

"It's really been very frustrating in a sense because I think sexually it turns him on: He likes it . . . [but I] just feel that sex is quite a trial because [I] can't get comfortable. . . . And I feel guilty about it because after all *his* hormones haven't changed!" (Pregnant mother interviewed in Ann Oakley's *Becoming a Mother.*)

"I want to have orgasm without foreplay three or four times everyday. I look at your father slyly, passively. I insist he come back to bed 'now.' . . . I am without shame. Never have I been in such sexual heat. Is this natural in pregnancy?" (Phyllis Chesler, in *With Child,* her pregnancy journal.)

There is quite a bit of variation in women's views toward intercourse during pregnancy. Men differ, also, some finding the pregnant body a turn-off, others finding it exciting. It is never easy to generalize about sexuality, and this nine-month period is no exception.

On the other hand, listing the few medical restrictions is easy.

▶ There are no restrictions on sex in the first trimester, unless there are medical concerns about miscarriage or signs of miscarriage. However, the woman may not be interested, due to fatigue or nausea. (In any trimester, the signs of miscarriage include bleeding from the vagina, vaginal or abdominal pain, rupture of the bag of waters. In these cases, the woman should refrain from intercourse and see her physician.)

▶ The second trimester is one of increased blood flow to the pelvis and vagina and elevated estrogen production. Women sometimes feel sexually supercharged at this time. There is no danger of hurting the fetus and no restrictions on sexual activity, except as noted above.

▶ In the third trimester, sex becomes awkward, especially in the traditional position. Other positions might be tried in which the man's weight does not rest on the woman's abdomen. Some doctors prefer that the couple be abstinent for the last four to six weeks, for fear of infection. Whether infection actually results from late intercourse has never been proven, however, except when the membranes (amniotic sack) had ruptured.

Some home-birth-oriented mothers actually use intercourse to start labor. "My husband and I took a long walk. I drank a tea made of cohosh, an herb used by the Indians to speed delivery. . . . We also made love. These three factors, combined with the readiness of the child to be born, produced a flash delivery. After less than an hour's intense labor, I gave birth to a girl at home (as planned)." This is Pippa Gordon's account of the birth of her second child, when she was thirty-five.

In short, intercourse can't hurt the baby, unless something else is wrong. For example, a woman who has had a series of miscarriages would probably be forbidden to have intercourse (she might also be confined to bed). But no one needs to practice abstinence because something *might* be wrong. Intercourse during pregnancy is permissable and enjoyable, between consenting adults, in ways that feel comfortable for both.

IN CONCLUSION

The adaptations to pregnancy are the beginning of motherhood. Pregnancy challenges the woman's assumptions and habits in many areas of life, and motherhood further changes and disrupts those assumptions and habits. As we've seen, older mothers have an advantage here. Success with prior crises is good preparation for coping with motherhood.

Knowing that every aspect of life will be affected, a little forethought and some self-understanding will help make every aspect of your life enriched.

Life with
a New Baby:
Up from Crisis

The focus of this chapter is not primarily child care or child development, but rather what happens to the over-thirty woman, her husband, and her life when the nurse puts a baby in her arms and says, "Congratulations, good luck—and good-bye!"

The arrival of a first baby presents a crisis for any family, but it is particularly significant for the older woman. Almost every aspect of her life is in a constant state of flux and reassessment for the first few weeks. Her previous ordered and predictable routine is on twenty-four-hour red alert. This chapter covers those first crucial weeks: decisions about baby care, life as a new mother, and finding your own parenting style.

Since all the fuss starts with the newborn, it seems appropriate to meet your baby, first.

MEET YOUR BABY

The first three months of the baby's life are called the "fourth trimester." This is the time when the infant

141

changes from being driven by inner needs and reflexes to being responsive to the outside world. Many people are familiar with the giggling five-month-old baby, playing with his toes and cooing. That sort of smiling baby is what the advertisements show, and it is what most people think of when they say "a baby."

But that is an older baby. The advertisements wouldn't dare show a newborn. Newborns don't laugh and coo. They cry or grimace or sleep; they don't smile.

They don't play with their toes or look at the mobile either. When awake, they often thrash around in a way that seems most uncontrolled. Arm movements are jerky, and they hit their faces with their hands and scratch themselves up with their fingernails. They don't seem to notice. One father was convinced that his healthy newborn had cerebral palsy; another mother was certain that her baby had been nerve-poisoned by the weed-control chemicals used on her neighbor's lawn. If a person expects a smiling, responsive baby, newborns can seem damaged.

Newborns aren't damaged, but they are very limited. Some newborns, the "good babies," sleep a lot. Others cry a lot instead. Even when they sleep, babies may or may not choose to do so at appropriate times (at night for example).

One mother described her reaction to nighttime feeding! "Before I had my baby, I had heard about the 2:00 A.M. feeding. I wasn't really too worried, though, about losing sleep. So you wake up at 2:00 A.M. and feed the baby. How long can that take, after all? Then you go back to bed. That's what I thought people meant by 2:00 A.M. feeding. I really wasn't prepared. She would go to bed around 10:00 P.M., sleep about three and a half, maybe four hours, wake up at 2:00, just like they said, and stay awake, eating or fussing or having a bowel movement or crying or burping and eating again until about 5:30 in the morning. She didn't just do this once. She did this regularly, about every other night, for the first six weeks of her life."

The behavior described above, unfortunately, is normal baby behavior. All newborns go through nights like that, some more than others. Some babies have it worse. They have colic.

Colic is loud, unexplained crying, which is generally assumed to come from digestive upset in the baby. Newborn babies have digestive systems that are not fully developed. Their tendency to spit up is just an outward symptom of the great inner disorganization. For example, in the first days of life, they go through something called "gut closure," in which the lining of their intestines changes permeability.

Of course, babies are organized enough to survive, and they do digest most of their food. But their digestive systems often have start-up problems, as you would expect from so complicated a chemical process. It actually takes a few weeks for most of the systems to switch over from intrauterine living to life outside.

In brief, newborns are seldom happy. They cry and fuss before, after, and between feedings. Gradually, however, they grow in their ability to focus on the world and watch their mother's face. They begin to smile. Sandra Scarr, in *Mother Care, Other Care,* describes the baby's first few weeks as "subcortical." She means that the higher level of the brain, the cortex, is not developed in newborns. Later, as the brain develops, dendrite (nerve fibers) begin to grow, the cortex expands, and less instinctive, more elaborate behaviors can be learned. As Scarr puts it, "By about six weeks of age, at the dawning of the dendrites, babies begin to smile at human faces and other interesting objects."

The growth of these abilities, the humanizing of the baby, is very exciting to watch. But at the beginning, newborns are rather crabby souls, and they aren't capable of giving the mother much positive feedback.

The Newborn's List of Talents

- Breathing. Babies are very good at breathing, and there is little need to worry that they will stop. Yes, there is something called sudden infant death syndrome (SIDS), and babies do die of it. But it is really quite rare and seems to be based on insufficiencies in the breathing-control center of the afflicted babies. It happens most often during the winter months, to babies between two and four months old, who are the children of young and poor mothers. Your new baby is not in the most vulnerable group. Not much is known about SIDS, but the occurrence of this problem seems to have nothing to do with how parents handle the baby, or whether they put him in a crib face up or face down.

All babies can avoid smothering. They can lift their heads enough to move their heads sideways if put nose down on a smooth surface. They don't need pillows, so a smooth surface is what they are usually on. They can bat a soft object away from their nose, even with their uncoordinated hand motions. Their gag reflex is very strong: they have less chance of choking on mucus or water than you do. Babies will keep breathing.

- Eating. The baby has a rooting reflex to help her find the nipple. If you stroke the side of her cheek, the infant will turn her head in the direction of the stroke, open her mouth, and start to grope. Her sucking reflexes are also well in place. Although early feeding may involve some difficulties, such as digestive upsets, these problems are unlikely to be caused by an unwillingness to suck. Infants even dream about nursing, as you can readily confirm by watching a newborn's mouth during sleep.

- Trying to hang on if there is a loud noise or sudden motion (Moro reflex). The baby startles: He throws out his arms and legs, cries out, and then brings together his arms and legs and grasps. If you think of a small animal falling out of a tree and alerting its mother to its plight, this reflex is easy to understand. This is why, incidentally, you are advised to support the infant's head: The baby's neck muscles are weak, and an unsupported head drops back. The infant perceives this as "sudden motion," which triggers the Moro reaction. He grabs out and starts to cry.

- **Observing.** Research has shown that a new baby can focus its eyes and look at things for as much as a minute or two at a time. Babies especially like to see smiling human faces. Luckily, mothers and fathers like to look at their baby's face, so every body gets some practice.

  But the research on a newborn's powers of observation should be taken as a guide, not a promise. In other words, since you know your baby can observe things, however briefly, watch for that behavior and encourage it. But don't expect looking around to be the newborn's main occupation. It isn't. That is why it was necessary to engage in all that research to discover that babies could focus.

- **Excreting (of course).** A newborn's stool changes color and consistency over the first few days: Your pediatrician will be able to inform you which color (green, yellow, brown) is appropriate at which time. This is all part of the baby's digestive start-up. Also, the baby's reaction to the uncomfortable feeling of "I have to make a bowel movement" is a good example of how much she is ruled by her inner drives. Every new mother has attempted to comfort an infant's strained cries, only to discover that the baby was merely getting ready to move her bowels. The baby *was* uncomfortable, but there was really nothing mother could do to help her.

The trouble is, for a new mother, those first six weeks before the dendrites dawn can seem endless. It is important to know that the baby's unhappiness is not your fault, and that you cannot ensure a happy two-week-old, no matter how hard you try. This section on the newborn is not really meant to be a treatise on infant development (see the bibliography for recommended reading on this subject), but to inform you enough about your infant to help you adapt to your life as a new mother.

Checklist: Calming a New Baby

▶ While he's crying, you might as well change his diapers. That's probably not the problem, but you wouldn't want to get him calmed down and asleep, only to remember he hadn't been changed for hours.

▶ Then try nursing him. Many new babies need to nurse a lot. Some may need to nurse twice, for forty-five minutes each time, in the space of two hours. After all that exertion, the baby may sleep several hours. Don't withhold nursing simply because you're thinking, "He can't be hungry, he just ate an hour ago." Never underestimate the disorganization of a newborn's digestive tract!

▶ A change in position can be a great help. Babies like to be held straight up, looking over your shoulder. It's not clear whether burping them or simply holding them upright is what causes the baby to calm down. Don't worry if she doesn't burp. Is she happier?

▶ A mother's heartbeat is a great soother. Try holding the baby close or in an infant carrier pack on your chest; then walk around.

▶ Rhythmic noises that imitate the human heart can also soothe a baby's soul. One mother put her baby in its infant seat on top of the clothes dryer. Then she put a tennis shoe and a towel in the dryer and turned it on (no heat; she didn't want to burn the tennis shoe). The vibration and muffled thumping calmed her baby "like magic."

▶ The vibration of a buggy or car ride may quiet your baby.

▶ Nursing doesn't always help, and sometimes babies need to suck, even when full. *Pacifier* isn't a dirty word. All the detrimental effects of pacifiers (potential problems with buck teeth and so on) have to do with an older child's use of a pacifier. For a baby under six months old, pacifiers are fine.

▶ Some babies like to be held so that they can "walk" on a hard surface.

▶ Another nice position for a baby is "swimming baby" —face down and held under the tummy. They like to practice holding their head up in this position for a short time. But if you do this too long, neck muscles will tire, and the baby will cry.

▶ Babies try very hard to watch children. Invite some children over to play with the baby (under your close supervision, of course).

▶ Rocking and singing sometimes helps.

▶ Some babies work themselves frantic and make their mothers frantic too. The mother tries everything, the baby still screams. The mother gets more upset, and the baby catches her mood. A vicious cycle. Break the cycle by putting the baby down in his crib, setting the kitchen minute minder for five or ten minutes, and using that time to try and collect yourself. After ten minutes, the baby may have fallen asleep; if that's not the case, he may now be ready to be soothed by something that didn't work earlier.

▶ Don't forget sickness. It's easy to blame your own mothering ability when in fact the baby should see the doctor about an ear infection. Be especially aware of sudden changes in your baby's disposition. Also, any fever in a brand-new baby is always cause for medical attention.

▶ Look for a "hot line" resource, someone to call when all else fails. This can be a professional community service or a trusted friend or relative. A tired, distracted mother deserves a friendly person just to listen, and maybe even to give advice.

LIFE AS A NEW OLDER MOTHER

"Before I had a baby, I was often rather scornful of the mothers I knew. They seemed to be making such obvious mistakes in raising their children. Now I see things differently. A lot differently. At least they kept the baby alive and healthy the first few months. Nobody can possibly know how much work that is until she's done it.

"About two weeks after the baby was born, I looked at myself in the mirror. I was absolutely white with fatigue; I looked like the hostage in one of those news reports: 'Mad gunman finally releases hostage after three days of police negotiations.' My face was full of pimples, my hair was falling out. I thought: 'You're a wreck; motherhood has wrecked you.' Just three weeks before the baby was born, I had made a presentation to one of the vice-presidents and his staff. I couldn't believe I had ever been organized and self-confident enough to do such a thing. Was I really once in a business maternity suit, makeup in place, very crisp and well prepared? At that point I went on my first crying jag. I felt that motherhood had ruined me."

Motherhood can be a very enriching experience from the point of view of the mother's maturity and self-knowledge. Unfortunately, maturity and self-knowledge don't come cheaply. Or as one woman said, "Don't tell me this is going to be another learning experience. I just hate learning experiences." Or, as another woman said, "Parenthood is a lesson in your limits."

The older mother can be especially shocked at the intensity of her reactions to the new situation. She is often used to succeeding, to having her world more or less under control. Self-confidence, that's an advantage of maturity. The disadvantage of maturity is that her self-expectations may be unrealistically high. As the lawyer in Chapter 1 said, "I know that if I had children, I could be a perfect mother." Not many women, young or old, would put it so bluntly. But many older women have highly idealized views of themselves as mothers.

Then they meet the baby. As described in the section above, a newborn is more in touch with its own bowels than with anything its mother does. To constantly tend someone who never says thank-you or even smiles is not necessarily very pleasant.

And of course, while this is going on, the mother is also losing sleep and recovering from childbirth. Her hormonal balance is changing, which may mean pimples, temporary hair loss, and depression. Her body still looks mildly pregnant. Extreme frustration is common, perhaps even expected. Simply continuing to function may feel like a major victory on some days. Sometimes just crying is an appropriate response to the environment.

We are emphasizing negative emotions here, because these are the ones that cause trouble. Descriptions of new motherhood that explain how wonderful it is going to be can leave the new mother feeling guilty as well as frustrated. But we must emphasize that the emotions of the first few weeks aren't all negative. One mother put it this way: "I could have spent all day just staring at the baby. I kept thinking, how perfect she is, how beautiful. It is hard to believe that she came out of my body." Infants bring joy as well as problems. We're trying to help the new mother deal with the problems. She's on her own with the joy.

Coping with the Big Four

There are four major aspects to the new-mother crisis. Being aware of them will not eliminate the problems, but may help turn them into challenges, rather than overwhelming and permanent changes to your life.

1. Fatigue. Recovering from pregnancy and birth would take some time even if the baby slept through the night immediately. But the baby doesn't sleep through the night immediately, and neither does the mother. Being chronically tired could depress anybody.

Many new mothers spend an extraordinary amount of psychic energy blaming themselves. *I'm home all day,* they think, *I really should be able to get a decent dinner on the table, write the thank-you notes for the baby presents, read that report my boss gave me.* The reason that new mothers aren't cooking, writing, reading is not laziness. It is fatigue and other demands on your time.

2. Frustration. If babies behaved all their lives the way that they behave as newborns, nobody would have them. Luckily, they improve. As an analogy, think of the first trimester of pregnancy, with all the nausea, fatigue, and ambivalence. At that point, you may well have hung on just because the second trimester was coming. Well, hang on with a newborn because, promise, the smiling Gerber baby really is just around the corner. Older babies (four months or so) are practically smiling machines. The second trimester of parenthood can be very pleasant.

3. Learning a new job without benefit of training. Despite her inexperience, the mother has many decisions to make: bottle or breast; pacifier or no pacifier; disposable or washable diapers; letting the baby cry for a few minutes as he is dropping off to sleep or rocking him asleep. If she believes some psychologists, each decision she makes is absolutely crucial to the child's development. Good intentions don't count; she is supposed to do it right. But she's tired and uncertain, and the baby isn't happy (after all, he's learning a new job too: living outside the womb). How can she do it right?

4. Self-expectations. From being an active woman, competent at her job and mistress of her house, as well as busy in the world of adults, she has changed. She's home with the baby, both of them tired and crabby, and she's not even able to meet the baby's demands. Being constantly at the beck and call of an infant is very wearing ("Your ears get tired, listening for the next cry," one mother said). If she is nursing, constantly exposing her breast to the baby may be subtly embarrassing (What if someone comes to the door?) and certainly, spending all that time sitting nursing the baby can't be right, can it? What happened to the woman who used to be in charge of her life and had the respect of adults at home and at work?

These concerns are not due to hysteria or lack of "mother instinct" or the possibility that you really shouldn't have had the baby. They are real problems, and part of their solutions lies in reevaluating your own expectations. Reevaluation won't solve all the problems: It won't make a newborn smile or relieve gas in a colicky infant. But reevaluation helps you keep your perspective on the situation.

First, forget the Chinese peasant "legend" that women just have a baby in the fields and go right back to hoeing. It isn't true. Every culture protects the rest and privacy of the new mother and baby. Among the Chinese, new mothers are encouraged to stay in bed, not sent out to do fieldwork. They are supposed to eat only warm food, since cold food is considered dangerous to a new mother in her fragile condition, and they are not supposed to receive any bad news.

Here in the United States, you will be happier if you realize that taking care of a new baby is among the hardest work anyone in the world can do. Every kind of stress is present. It is unrealistic to expect that you'll go through the day cheery and humorous. It is even unrealistic to expect you'll make dinner.

This is the time for hired help or take-out food. This is the time for doing the laundry but for forgetting the other housework (or hiring someone else to do it, if it bothers you). Reduce your self-expectations. If nursing the baby takes many hours a day, do it. Somebody else can make dinner, but who else do you know who is lactating? Who else in the family just went through childbirth? Give yourself a break.

If you can forgive yourself for the fact that not everything is running smoothly, it will help you emphasize the good moments (new babies have the sweetest odor, and the nicest little hands that can grip your finger!) and deemphasize the bad moments. The big four won't be so big anymore.

It is also most important to realize that individual decisions about baby care are not all that crucial. This seems to be easier for younger mothers, who "kind of expect" the baby will be all right. For older mothers, used to turning in perfect reports and well educated on psychological theory, insecurities are often greater. But remember, *because* you are a mature woman you are more likely to correctly read your baby's signals and do what is right for her (see research reported in Chapter 1). What you need is some guidance on decisionmaking (see discussion below) to free yourself of that anxiety, so that you can enjoy your baby.

After all, no scientific study has ever shown that babies given pacifiers turn out badly. Diapers are really a matter of doing what is easiest and what you can afford. Breastfeeding is a splendid way to feed a baby (see the section on breast and bottle, below). But nothing will guarantee psychological health for the baby. Moreover, babies are different in their demands, and thus some of your decisions will be made for you—by the baby himself.

In short, there are no guarantees, no matter what you do. And there is no evidence that any reasonable, well-meaning decision will have bad consequences.

DECISIONS: BREAST OR BOTTLE?

Although this section describes the advantages of breastfeeding and gives advice for successful nursing, that doesn't mean that babies should be raised only at the breast. Most bottle-fed babies grow into happy adults. Nor does breastfeeding solve all medical and psychological problems. There used to be infant mortality back in the days when all babies were breastfed. As for the psychological advantages, we must remember that Caligula and Attila the Hun were undoubtedly breastfed.

Also, some mothers simply don't want to nurse their babies. They may feel embarrassed, since in this country breasts are regarded as practically a genital organ. Because of this, some women only feel comfortable nursing in extreme privacy. Others find the idea of putting a baby to the breast disgusting. Hugh Hefner may be partially to blame, but the attitudes were there before he exploited them.

If the idea of nursing makes you personally uncomfortable, don't feel bad about it. Nursing or bottle-feeding are just one aspect of child care. The ability to breastfeed is not some miraculous touchstone for determining fitness for motherhood. If you have strong negative feelings about breastfeeding, please skip the next five subsections. They are intended to help nursing mothers and possibly convince the uncertain. They are not intended to make bottle-feeding mothers feel guilty. There is too much guilt in motherhood already.

Older mothers, however, are usually quite successful at nursing babies. They tend to be more relaxed about their sexuality, and less tense or embarrassed by breastfeeding. Jane, a leader in La Leche League, the national nursing mothers support organization, notes that older mothers often have more patience and perseverance than younger women and are less discouraged by small problems at the beginning. They also take the health advantages of nursing more seriously: Breastfeeding helps prevent allergies, and that often matters more to an older mother who has seen a friend chauffeuring the children off to the allergist. "One older mother in my group came from an allergic family and was allergic herself. Even though she went back to work earlier than I would have recommended, she kept the baby on breast milk for a year, and successfully avoided allergies to cow's milk and other foods for the child."

The Advantages of Nursing

The advantages of breastfeeding your baby are threefold: nutritional advantages for the baby, psychological advantages for the baby, and psychological advantages for the mother.

Nutritional Advantages for the Baby

Breast milk is the perfect food for babies. For newborns, who cannot digest milk because they are still undergoing gut closure, the breasts make colostrum. This fluid, which contains antiviral antibodies, will protect the infant from disease for six months, even if breast-feeding is not continued. (Bottle-fed babies get sugar water at this time, which provides energy but no disease protection.)

After two to five days, when the milk comes into the breasts, almost 100 percent of its protein is digestible. The protein in cow's milk, however, forms large curds, which are difficult for the baby to digest, and so about 50 percent of the protein in formula is excreted. In addition, the foreign proteins in cow's milk sometimes provoke cow's-milk allergies, which might have been prevented if the same proteins were introduced later in the child's life.

Formula and breast milk usually have the same amount of simple sugars. But the bottle-fed baby actually gets more sugars per ounce of digested protein than the breastfed baby gets, because of incomplete digestion. This may tend to make him obese. At the age of six months, bottle-fed babies usually weigh more than breastfed babies do.

Formula contains the same amount of fat as breast milk, but formula is homogenized, giving the baby the same amount of fat with each swallow. Mother's milk isn't homogenized. First, protein-rich milk comes down from the breast; later in the nursing the breasts release the fat-rich milk. So the baby gets his rich "dessert" only if he drinks off all the first milk. A bottle-fed baby gets the same amount of fat at each sip, and he may "fill up" on his calorie needs before having taken in the appropriate amount of nutrition.

Since no human antibodies occur in formula, formula-fed babies have somewhat higher susceptability to infections than nursed babies do. With modern antibiotics available, this is less important than it used to be.

Scientists have not yet discovered all the ways that mother's milk adapts to and meets the baby's needs, but it is well known that breast milk prevents allergies and illness. Nutritionally, then, breast is best.

Psychological Advantages for the Baby

Now we're treading on dangerous ground. There is absolutely no evidence that nursed babies grow into emotionally healthier adults. Nevertheless, the process of nursing tends to be very soothing to babies. Where a baby will pull away from a bottle and scream because he is full, he will keep nursing at an empty breast, getting just a small trickle of milk, until he falls asleep. While the bottle-fed baby receives what his mother measures out, the breastfed baby regulates his own nursing.

A nursing baby is in a partnership with the mother. He must learn to suck in a way that stimulates his mother's let-down reflex. (Without a let-down reflex, milk would constantly drip from the mother's breasts as it was produced. Instead, it stays up in the breast until the baby's sucking triggers the hormones that signal to let the milk down.) Sucking for a moment or two, without much reward until the milk lets down, teaches the baby a little patience and a little trust.

There is absolutely no evidence that any of this early learning has any long-term effect on the child's personality. But mothers who have nursed babies feel that it does. They feel that being part of a nursing team helped calm their babies, and it helped the mothers to have a close and warm relationship with their child.

Psychological Advantages for the Mother

Let's look at evolution for a moment. How did nature ensure that babies would get nursed? By making it pleasant for the mother.

There are two major hormones that control this pleasure. One is prolactin, which regulates the milk supply. You might call this the maternal hormone: If you inject prolactin into male animals or never-pregnant females, they suddenly get quite solicitous of the young.

When prolactin is on your side, taking care of the baby is easier. It is also an antidepressant. Women who wean their babies feel depressed partially because they no longer produce this hormone.

The second hormone is oxytocin, which is released when the milk lets down. Women also release this hormone at orgasm. In nursing, it is not felt as strongly as it is in orgasm; instead, it acts as a tranquilizer. "A flood of peace and joy" is how one mother described the feeling of letting down the milk. "I'm an oxytocin addict," said another mother. "All my life, I saw the world as push, push, push. When I nurse the baby, I just feel so at peace, as if everything I've ever done is right."

Her feelings are reflected in the attitudes of other nursing mothers. Sara Winter did a study of the psychology of nursing mothers. She showed them various "action pictures" while they were breastfeeding their babies. She showed the same pictures to a control group of mothers who had weaned their babies. The nursing mothers had very positive, very calm things to say about the pictures. For example, if shown a trapeze artist, nursing mothers said nothing about danger. Instead they discussed the joy of flying through the air, followed by the safety of grabbing the partner's hands. The other mothers were more realistic, but the nursing mothers had a more positive attitude.

The nursing mother has hormones on her side for those crucial first weeks of parenting. She has a maternal-feeling hormone, prolactin, and a tranquilizer, oxytocin. New babies are a big strain, so evolution and hormones provide the nursing mother with a little help in the beginning days.

Nursing for Novices

Starting to nurse is not easy. (Is anything about beginning motherhood easy?) Nursing mothers, especially, need expert advice. In her book, *The Tender Gift*, Dana Raphael points out that you cannot predict who will be successful at nursing by asking if the mother shows a strong desire to nurse. The crucial factor is not her desire, but rather the availability of someone knowledgable to help and advise her.

Many women in this country have never even seen a nursing baby. It is definitely best to get some help. La Leche League has many experienced nursing mothers happy to give practical advice.

Later in nursing, things are much easier. After the baby is four months old, he usually starts on solid foods. After that, nursing becomes as much a comfort as a source of nutrition. As Karen Pryor explains in *Nursing Your Baby*, it is easier to work and nurse the older baby than to work and bottle feed. The baby nurses cozily in the morning, again when Mom comes home, and at bedtime. The availability of his old comfort makes him happier and less demanding in the evening, and the nursing hormones relax the mother after her tense day.

Nursing Is a State of Mind: Advice on Bottle-Feeding

As one doctor said, "Nursing is a state of mind as much as a physical act. You can be a 'nursing mother' and bottle feed." However, bottle feeding is also fraught with uncertainty for a new mother.

A bottle-feeding mother commented: "I wish there were a La Leche League for us bottle-feeders. I hate to call my doctor all the time, but sometimes I don't know what to do. All kinds of bottles, all kinds of nipples, including one that is supposed to prevent orthodontic problems later, different formulas. Good Lord! Every time my newborn cried, I wondered if I had made the right choice." In the first few weeks, when the newborn cries, the breast-feeding mother often blames herself (wasn't nursing supposed to cure everything?), and the bottle-feeding mother thinks she should switch formulas. Nobody seems to want to admit that things can be tough the first few weeks, no matter what you do.

But you can do a few things to make bottle-feeding more like nursing. Let's start with the nipple you choose. Not being pediatricians or orthodontists, we don't plan to give advice on exactly which nipple is best. But we can advise you to make sure the nipple has a nice, slow rate of flow, so that the baby doesn't take her milk too quickly. All babies need sucking practice. Even though it seems convenient, you don't actually want to feed the baby in five minutes.

Breastfed babies may nurse for twenty to forty minutes a feeding at first; try to be sure that the bottle-fed infant will need to take twenty minutes to finish. The nipple hole should let milk drip slowly when the bottle is held upside down. The nipple should be relatively loosely attached to the bottle. With most bottles, if air can't get in, the infant can't get milk out.

Then there is holding. Hold your baby close while feeding her. As a matter of fact, try to hold the baby in a mock breastfeeding position, with the head somewhat raised, which keeps her closer to where she can hear a heartbeat. Some doctors also think that feeding a baby while she is flat on her back predisposes the child to ear infections.

Never prop a bottle, either. Babies need some human contact. Take the time to hold her. Propping a bottle tends to be habit forming; pretty soon you find yourself putting the baby to sleep while she holds her own bottle. And soon after that, you find yourself taking the baby to the dentist with "bottle-baby cavities," because milk in the mouth at night rots teeth.

Obesity can be a problem with bottle-fed babies. An infant finishing a bottle may give the mother a nice sense of completion, but more calories may have been taken in than was necessary. Don't urge your baby to drink more than is clearly wanted.

If you did choose to bottle-feed, your husband (or someone else) can help you with all aspects of baby care. As a matter of fact, he can do half the work. The question is, will he? Will the work be divided fifty-fifty?

ON DUTY/OFF DUTY: CONTINUOUS COVERAGE FOR THE BABY

Before a baby is born, the working couple's life can be described as an alliance. She does what she wants, he does what he wants, and some of the time they do things together. After the baby is born, husband and wife suddenly become partners in a very demanding continuous-coverage system.

Continuous coverage is how police departments and hospitals are run, where problems come up around the clock. In the newborn's at-home continuous-coverage system, however, there aren't enough workers for three shifts. The baby needs tending twenty-four hours a day, but mother and father are usually the only ones around to provide it.

This new situation changes their marriage from the laissez-faire alliance it was before the baby. Now, one is on duty while the other is off. The need for continuous coverage has several unsettling effects on a marriage. For example, in the book *Transition to Parenthood*, Ralph and Maureen LaRossa describe a marriage in which there had been many conflicts about household responsibility before the baby was born. Although the couple had these disagreements, they enjoyed each other's company and took a lot of pleasure in shared activities, such as the theatre group in which they were both active.

After the baby was born, the husband returned to the theatre group, and the wife stayed home. Each blamed the other. He felt she was trying to control him, to make him as house-bound as she was. She felt he was running away from his responsibilities. Some of the couple's postbaby interviews with the LaRossas ended with the wife leaving the room in tears.

This is not a good example of how to negotiate coverage after a baby is born. As a matter of fact, it is a very poor example of how to run a marriage. Unfortunately, it is not really very extreme, except that the conflict took place around a theatre group, when usually it takes place about the man's job. As one woman said, "It's very fashionable around here for men to be with their wives at the Lamaze classes, be there at the birth, take a few days off, and all that. They are very proud of their role as coaches and really feel their wives couldn't have given birth without their presence. Three weeks after the birth, it is fashionable for them to be back at work, working late, acting as if nothing had happened."

Most men's involvement with their children goes beyond fashion. But this woman had a point. Men are expected to be back at work, and back completely, very quickly. Four weeks later, the baby may not be sleeping through the night, but the husband is supposed to be.

The LaRossas illustrated the differences in society's expectations by their interviews with a more enlightened couple. This couple had a strong and resilient marriage, and were committed to equality between men and women. They both worked at a university and had somewhat flexible hours. He was a professor, she a lecturer-instructor (nontenured faculty). After the baby was born, they made a conscious effort to split the child care. He stayed home with the baby three mornings a week while she taught. He also took care of the baby various evenings, while she went to meetings. He was the only man among the couples the LaRossas interviewed who really took care of the infant, for several hours at a time, on a regular basis. Husband and wife both felt that the baby had deepened and enriched their love for each other.

But all was not as equal as it seemed on the surface. The wife took care of the baby far more hours than the husband did. When he spoke of his child-care involvement, he spoke of "good mornings" and "bad mornings." During a "good morning," the baby slept a lot, and he was able to get his own work done. He only had to really tend to the baby's needs for about an hour, until his wife came home. On "bad mornings," the baby didn't sleep much. On those mornings, he wasn't able to get much of his work done. Eventually, "bad" mornings replaced "good" mornings when the baby gave up his morning nap. The couple then hired a baby-sitter for those mornings when the wife worked. The husband really did not feel that he could be responsible for child care at the cost of his job advancement.

As the LaRossas commented: "Before the transition to parenthood, it is easy for couples . . . to believe that they are nontraditional." The LaRossas' work showed that, even in the most concerned households, husband and wife don't split the baby care fifty-fifty. (No couples where the wife went to work and the husband stayed home were interviewed, however.) Other studies also show the man doing far less housework or baby care than his wife does. There is no 50-percent solution. As the LaRossas point out, the larger culture, with its expectations, does not really allow equality of child care.

With this given, it is simply our purpose in this chapter to help loving and well-meaning couples think about dividing the work of parenting in a mutually satisfactory way. The first step is to realize the strains that being on call twenty-four hours a day puts on the couple. If not handled thoughtfully, the situation can become a "zero sum game": Whenever one person wins, the other loses. In the case of parents of a new baby, the prize in the game is free time.

The solution to this problem is twofold. First, the father must realize that if the mother is on twenty-four-hour coverage without definite relief periods that she can look forward to, she will have problems being a good mother. Unrelieved coverage is what the single mothers were talking about when they said, "You can go crazy." Unrelieved coverage is too much for most people to take emotionally. If faced with such a situation, most people will rely on psychological distancing mechanisms to save their sanity. They will be physically there for the baby but emotionally divorced.

In short, the father can save his wife's sanity and maintain the quality of his child's care by taking on a specified amount of baby care each day, perhaps two hours each evening. Yes, this can even be done if the mother is nursing. No nursed baby ever died of starvation if the mother went out for a few hours to shop with a friend or to see a movie, or else stayed home and just read a book in peace. Other couples switch nights: his night on, her night off.

Taking over for two hours a day or for alternate evenings is also the best thing a father can do for his own relationship with the child. Fathers who are basically visitors, just putting in a few minutes of occasional play with the child, rather quickly get out of touch with the child's signals. The mother becomes the official interpreter of the child's behavior; the father, a mystified observer of her seemingly miraculous knowledge. But the mother's knowledge of the baby doesn't spring from some sacred maternal source. Her knowledge of the baby's moods simply comes from hour-by-hour responsibility. Hour-by-hour responsibility by the father will give him the same knowledge, as well as similar empathy with the child.

The second part of the solution comes in recognizing that the husband and wife will almost certainly not do equal amounts of baby care, except in those households that have complete role reversal. Most families become more patriarchal in the first few months after the baby is born. The mother is tied up with the baby, and she is not earning as much money. The father is less tied down and still working. Power follows money, and freedom of action follows power. Power shifts to the man.

The man and woman can have arguments about this, if they wish. Or they can accept that this situation is temporary. They can realize that this restructuring occurs in almost every family (for a while) after the birth of the first baby. If nothing else, people fall back on their old role models, their own parents, when they are unsure of what to do. You should realize that you have not been deluded and seduced by a closet chauvinist: At no time in their lives will the constraints on the man's actions, and those on the woman's actions, feel and be so different. It hurts, but this extreme situation is only temporary.

Tips for Time-Sharing

▶ The father will not be as responsible for baby care as the mother is, unless the couple have complete role reversal. If husband and wife both accept this, life will be easier.

▶ The mother cannot be responsible for the baby twenty-four hours a day, or else the quality of her life and the quality of the child's care will decline together.

▶ There must be a set time—each evening, or every other evening—when the mother is off duty. Most evenings, the father will take over. Some days, they might arrange for a baby-sitter.

▶ The father's involvement on a day-to-day, full-responsibility basis will lead to benefits for him: a real understanding of his child and a strong relationship between them.

▶ Fathers and mothers should be flexible. A sick baby, for example, presents an emergency for which standard agreements give way.

REMEMBER LEISURE?

Couples without children participate in a wide variety of activities, many of which they greatly enjoy. After the baby comes, outside activities usually grind to a halt. Part of this is simple fascination with the baby: Nothing else seems as interesting. But the other part has to do with less cheerful issues. Mother is tired, she finds that baby-sitters are expensive, and she doesn't want to leave the baby for very long, especially if she's nursing. It just seems like a lot of trouble. This is an aspect of the choice you made to have a child, and it is a part of the natural evolution of your lives as parents. Involvement with the baby simply pushes aside many of your former activities.

Unfortunately, after three months of devoted parenting, "all the fun we used to have" can seem like a dream now gone forever, as baby takes up time, energy, and money. Even this good a thing can go too far, you discover. While older parents may be prepared for a major transition, it does nobody, including the baby, any good for the parents to entirely give up adult leisure activities. Frequently, the difficulty is simple timing. Many mothers feel uncomfortable if they are away from their babies for very long, especially if they are nursing. Father's suggestion that they spend this Saturday on the friend's boat is likely to be met with "Can we take Jennifer?" Such a question may well inspire an explosive reply.

The problem is that many mothers find it difficult to leave small babies for ten hours at a time. Their hormones make it difficult, especially if they are nursing and full of prolactin.

Of course, some mothers make an early decision not to be too involved with baby care. They hire live-in help and more or less go about their business. For the purposes of this chapter, however, we will continue to speak of the more usual case, in which the mother does not have live-in help. She has been primarily responsible for the baby for a few weeks, and her husband is urging her to take a break.

Though a full-day excursion may lead to conflict, most mothers thoroughly enjoy a two- or three-hour vacation from baby care. Therefore, frequent small breaks from the baby are a far better idea than occasional all-day outings. For half of the all-day outing, the mother's mind is likely to be elsewhere. For the full three hours, however, she will be able to concentrate on the father, as well as on having fun. If the mother is nursing, frequent small breaks are not only a better idea, they are the only idea. Mothers cannot leave nursing babies who are under three months old for more than a few hours, without making elaborate preparations (freezing milk, bringing along a breast pump to relieve the pressure, and so on).

It is probably best to begin going out with your husband but without the baby by the time the baby is five or six weeks old. Go to dinner, see a movie. Everybody in the family needs to know that the baby will survive for two hours in the mother's absence. The mother, especially, needs to be reminded of the outside world and of the adult activities in which she likes to participate.

Which brings us inevitably to the subject of sex. Intercourse in the first few weeks after childbirth can be uncomfortable for the mother or else expressly forbidden by her doctor. Foreplay with the woman's breasts may be constrained by leaking milk, which can embarrass both husband and wife. There is no real reason for embarrassment, but sometimes it may feel like the baby has truly taken over everything—including his mother's body.

And then, at least once, when man and woman are finally getting together for some shared enjoyment, the baby will wake up and begin to cry. For the mother this presents a classic role conflict: Should she ignore husband or baby? The husband may quite legitimately feel that he no longer has his wife's complete attention.

It turns out that sex is another area that lends itself to some renegotiation after childbirth. It presents another example of how the man's and woman's desires are no longer in the kind of equilibrium that was worked out before the baby. New mothers are frequently tired, as well as uncomfortable with their still-flabby and nursing bodies. The episiotomy (a surgical incision of the vaginal opening made by the doctor to facilitate the birth) may still hurt. But for the husband, renewing sexual intercourse with his wife is usually very important. Men don't have an easy time asking for reassurance, although they, too, need it in the early days. For most men, intercourse is more than simple relief of sexual tension; it is a way to know that they are loved and accepted.

Again, the solution is only understanding and time. When the child is a few months old and its sleeping patterns become more fixed, when the mother starts getting more sleep, then things will improve. When her body has completely recovered from childbirth, things will also get better. In the meantime, the man might just remember that the woman is more tired and uncomfortable than usual, and the woman might well remember that the man needs reassurance that he is still loved.

WHAT BABIES NEED: FINDING YOUR OWN PARENTING STYLE

Babies change with great rapidity. The baby who was oblivious to dirty diapers at two months may hate them at six months. The baby that didn't smile at four weeks will smile most of the time at four months. As one mother said: "No sooner did I get to know what to do, what her cries meant, than she changed signals on me."

This changing of signals also means constant regrouping on the part of the mother. Decisions aren't made just once; they are made over and over again as the baby grows and daily life changes. In order to make reasonable decisions and develop your own parenting style, it is worthwhile to know a little about how babies change and what they really need.

Touching is important. Babies like to be rocked and touched. Indeed, they cannot live without it, as orphanages early in this century proved conclusively. Touching is one of the most natural and enjoyable parts of baby care for both infants and parents.

Babies also need stimulation, a need that increases as the infant gets older. Luckily, appropriate amounts of stimulation are not hard to provide, especially at first. You don't need an infant gym to ensure your baby's healthy development. Newborn babies like to look at human faces, and most mothers and fathers like to look at babies.

Babies of less than three months old cannot be "spoiled." (The term *spoiled* is used here because it is the customary term for describing a demanding child. The idea that a baby or child becomes like a piece of moldy fruit is nevertheless disgusting.) The essence of "spoiling" is that the child remembers that something was done for him in the past and demands that same thing as his right in the future.

Until infants are around three months old, they don't

have enough brain development to be spoiled. They can't remember what happened last night and expect it again. They can be difficult, they can be hard to live with, but they cannot be "spoiled" until they have some sort of memory. Anything you can do to keep a young infant happy is quite all right.

On the other hand, older babies can be "spoiled." After babies are three months old, they have enough memory to begin to expect things. Sometimes the baby can expect things that it may be inconvenient for the parents to provide.

Note that it is the inconvenience to the parents rather than the expectations of the baby that determine whether the child is considered "spoiled" or not. For example, one mother found that she could put her baby to sleep by walking with him for a few minutes after giving him his evening bottle. Naturally, there was no lack of people to advise her that she had "spoiled" her baby, that he would always expect to be walked to sleep, and so on.

Nevertheless, she continued to walk him to sleep, because she did not feel particularly inconvenienced by the procedure. After all, he was always asleep in a short time. It fit in with her life. This was a clear case of "spoiled" being in the eye of the beholder. (Babies change so rapidly, by the way, that the walking-him-to-sleep routine lasted less than three months. So much for "always.")

Older babies can be encouraged and partially molded to fit in with the family. For example, at some point in their lives, most babies begin to take a late-afternoon nap. Some mothers object to this nap: A baby that slept from 4:00 to 6:00 P.M. is unlikely to go back to sleep before 10:00 or 11:00, robbing the mother of some quiet time in the evening.

The mothers who object quickly discover that they can keep the baby awake through the late-afternoon nap. At the risk of a having somewhat tired and crabby baby in the early evening, they can ensure that the child will go to bed by 8:00.

Other mothers let the child sleep in the afternoon and

fit her into the family's evening activities. These types of variations of baby care seem to have no ill effects on babies whatsoever. Such decisions are part of the emerging parenting style of the mother; they are part of the baby's learning to be a member of the family.

IN CONCLUSION

Over the first six months of your baby's life, he will change from a crabby creature ruled by his digestive system into a smiling, gurgling member of the family. The hours of the day and night will merge into each other at first, and then gradually differentiate themselves again. If you nurse the baby, you will find yourself sitting with him at the breast for long hours at first, and then less as the months go on.

The work of constantly taking care of the baby changes scope, and your division of labor with your husband will change also. The relationship will evolve from no sex and frantic nights with the baby, into more pleasant evenings.

You will get to know your own baby. Babies differ a lot. Some are active and hard to handle. Some are so easy and contemplative that the parents worry about retardation.

Will you be trying to stimulate a quiet baby? In his biography, Isaac Asimov describes the first year with his daughter: "Robyn, when she wasn't crying, lay there quietly and at peace. Which was fine, except that we would have welcomed some indication that she was making contact with the universe." (She turned out fine.)

Or will you be trying to calm an active baby? "First he had colic, then he took teething hard, then he started walking: running around the house, knocking himself against the furniture. He had stitches twice before he was two. Once, he literally ran full-tilt into a wall." (A man describing his son, who also turned out fine.)

The nature of your baby will influence your parenting style.

For the first few months, everything changes rapidly.

Decisions and revisions are made constantly. But at the end of those months, you know how to handle the baby you have. You have completed what one mother called "an introductory course in miracles." You have met many challenges, and you have a right to feel proud of yourself. You and your husband have worked out some mutually satisfactory arrangements for sharing child care. Furthermore, the baby is sleeping on a reasonable schedule, and life is becoming more orderly again.

Is it time to go back to work?

The Decision
to Return to Work

In a perfect world, we would clone ourselves. Then one part of us could be home, playing with the baby, while the other part was working, earning money, and getting promotions.

On the covers of magazines we can see pictures of women who supposedly have cloned themselves. Inside the magazine is an article about how having twins didn't slow her down a bit. The cover woman still made chairperson of the board, or founded a multimillion-dollar company, or starred in a movie, or wrote two best-selling books. She did it all, and at the same time continued being an excellent mother.

Of course, we don't know everything about these women, despite their media coverage. They are, for example, often reticent about divulging what kind of money they earn. But each reader of the magazine does know exactly how many hours superwoman gets in a day: twenty-four. And she has to allocate these hours to work and child care, just as any other working mother does.

One woman said: "As soon as I got pregnant, I was in a no-win situation. I either had an abortion, which a lot of people think is terrible; or had the baby and stayed home, meaning that someone else supports me, which many people think is parasitical and unliberated; or had the baby and went back to work, which many people think is inhuman and unmotherly." A bleak view of the situation, perhaps, but it is also a useful antidote to the view implied by those incredible women on magazine covers. After all, the root meaning of *incredible* is "not to be believed." It is time for a little reality.

THE REALITY OF THE BALANCING ACT

Most mothers have to go back to work. That is the reality of life in the 1980s. Having a baby is not (and financially cannot be) the signal for retirement. The question is when and how you, a unique and individual new mother, should arrange your own reentry.

The stereotype of the over-thirty, first-time mother is that of a well-paid professional woman, someone who can easily afford a housekeeper. To a certain extent, this stereotype bears itself out. At least, such a woman is more likely to be professional, if not necessarily well paid. According to the population bulletin "Delayed Childbearing in the U.S.: Facts and Fictions," over 50 percent of over-thirty, first-time mothers hold "professional" jobs. However, "professional" for women includes many relatively poorly paid careers, such as nurse, teacher, nutritionist, and social worker. Moreover, another 36 percent of older first-time mothers are not professional; they are sales, clerical, or service workers. Overall, among all workers, women employed full-time only earn fifty-nine cents for each dollar that full-time employed men earn.

Women must work within these financial limitations. It is not easy to finesse. Nor is it easy for us, as authors of this book, to offer advice on making certain choices, as if financial constraints did not exist, as if mothers usually got a few months' paid maternity leave, as if all mothers could all simply hire live-in help and go back to their exciting executive careers. So before we go on to helping individuals with their personal decisions, we'd like to comment on the general situation.

Placing Blame

Why is it so hard for women to decide when and how to go back to work after having a baby? And why is it so difficult for us to help women decide? It is because society puts mothers in a needlessly difficult situation and then blames them; it's a classic case of blaming the victim.

Sixty percent of the working mothers in this country get no paid maternity leave. The lucky ones get up to two months. In France, mothers get four months' paid leave; in Sweden, nine months; in England, four and a half months.

In the United States, it is completely up to the parents to finance the care of their children. Many other countries give families an allowance per child, which is then taken away from the rich in taxes. America doesn't do anything as egalitarian as that.

And even in the cases in which something is done for a working mother, the approach tends to be rather backhanded. Paid maternity leave, for example, is based on a mother's physical disability as she recovers from childbirth. It is explicitly *not* paid time off to get started in child-rearing. Adoptive mothers rarely get any time off, no matter how liberal a company's benefits policy is. Taking care of children is simply not a concern of employers.

Society's vision of the family, as reflected in legislation, seems to be based on the Dick-and-Jane readers of the '50s, when Daddy went to work and Mommy stayed home. The majority of our legislators consider themselves "profamily" if they support that sort of living arrangement, and somehow "antifamily" if they encourage an easier life for working women.

The world, however, is not the same as Dick's and Jane's. If every working mother quit work tomorrow, society would grind to a halt. Over 50 percent of married women are in the labor force. Over 50 percent of mothers of preschool children and 45 percent of the mothers of children under a year old are in the labor force. But if there is ever a conflict between work and taking care of a child, that problem is considered to be the mother's own unique burden.

Why do many companies allow for paid time off for military reserve service but not for taking a child to a doctor? Why is a few years in the military considered good training for job advancement and responsibility, but the same few years off for motherhood considered at best an inconvenient interruption? We are not antimilitary, but we wonder whether a society that can make some concessions in the work world because armies are important, might consider some changes because babies are important.

Society isn't going to change in the next few months, however, when you have to make your own decision. So, back to reality.

The Reality of Parenting

Why do women usually *want* to take more than a few weeks off to be with their babies? One reason is that the first few months of motherhood constitute an intense learning experience for a woman, an experience that is hard to interrupt. She is getting to know her baby and is adjusting to the role and demands of motherhood. She is beginning to figure out what makes the baby happy and watch, with great joy, his day-to-day progress.

She is also growing attached to her baby. "I wasn't sure I loved her until she was a couple of weeks old." Love, with babies or adults, does not usually strike at one blow. Mothers and fathers often believe that it should be love at first sight in the delivery room, but how can you truly love someone you've just met? There is relief, along with joy and fascination, in the delivery room. Love comes later.

The same is true of the baby. It is uncertain what the terms *love* or *attachment* would mean to a newborn. A newborn can recognize his mother by the particular smell of her body and can associate that odor with food and comfort; that is all the baby is capable of. Is it love? Not really.

It takes several months for a baby to really recognize its mother, and prefer Mommy in strange situations. The quality of the baby's security also varies. Babies whose mothers are good at "reading" the baby, responding appropriately to the baby's cries, seem to have a stronger trust in mother as a "safe base." Older mothers are particularly good at understanding their babies, as we noted in Chapter 1. Other studies, called "strange-situation experiments," also show that the babies of older, middle-class mothers tend to consider mother a "safe base" more often than babies of younger or poorer mothers do. They are "securely attached." Other babies, on the other hand, have a hard time adjusting to new situations, and aren't able to receive effective comfort from their mothers. These babies are called "anxiously attached," which is actually a pretty good description of the way they behave. For the mother, reading an infant's needs successfully implies being around the infant and learning to interpret her sounds and cries.

Loving the baby, growing attached, is one aspect of the reality of parenting. But it is not the only part. The average mother doesn't go around in a haze of developing love all day. After the trauma of the first few weeks, she has time to do other things: cook dinner, do the shopping, write the thank-you notes, watch the soap operas, get bored.

Babies are not perfect company. It is hard to discuss current events with a infant, and it is impossible for a baby to respond appropriately to even a very well-written memo. There is a great deal of dull, repetitive work in taking care of babies and small children. And then, the mother has lost a certain status in the home and outside, because she isn't working and earning money.

Speaking of money, the economic situation at home is certainly getting tight. All those expenses: the phone calls cross-country when the baby was born, the higher utility bills from all the laundry, the leftover part of the hospital bill that the insurance wouldn't pay. Will this family ever get out from under? Can this credit rating be saved?

Going back to work begins to look attractive. Money, adults to talk to, status in the eyes of your friends, a shift of power back in your direction vis-à-vis your husband. Who could ask for anything more?

The Reality of Working

Yes, it is possible to go back to work full time at two or six weeks after birth and still have a very well-cared-for baby: Just have live-in help. If someone else is taking care of the baby and the household, the mother can get back to her job as soon as she can recover from the physical trauma of birth.

Rich women have always had help. Nannies, governesses, maids (and, in the old days, wet-nurses) were always waiting in the wings. In the well-off household of a century ago, these hired women took on daily care of the child directly after the birth. Producing an heir was a mother's job; day-to-day child care was not.

Today, as in the past, if a mother is rich enough to afford live-in help and skilled enough to pick good people, children can be raised well by servants. Statesmen, poets, philosophers have been raised that way for hundreds of years, in manors and castles and elegant homes all over Europe. These children have cared about their mothers. They have differentiated between servants and parents. They may have had a great deal of affection for their old nannies, but they knew who their mothers were, and they loved them.

Many present-day executive women, and most of the women on the magazine covers, follow this old pattern. These are usually women who are very focused on their work and really cannot imagine taking any significant time away from their chosen profession. They also make enough money to hire competent help. As one executive said, "People ask me, 'How do you run your home, with three children, and also run your firm?' The answer is that I don't. We've always had a housekeeper; for a while we had a housekeeper and a nanny. I'm responsible for hiring these people, for making sure the house runs smoothly and the children are treated well, but I don't do it all. Nobody can."

But servants are not the reality for most working women. For them, the reality of going back to work is a rigid schedule, based on day-care availability, and an abrupt transition from being with the baby all day (until you are tired of the baby) to being with the baby only mornings and evenings (when you are just plain tired). It is a sudden interruption of the learning process of becoming a mother, and it is the beginning of a painful balancing act. How superwoman does it is not relevant.

So why do women go back to work? Generally, they do it for the money—that is, after all, why most women work. This does not mean that they are not also interested in their jobs or in advancement. Emphasis on the career aspects of work is very fashionable now, but few women are truly on the fast track to the stars. Many have satisfying jobs with some advancement potential, but these jobs do not pay in the six-figure range or the high five-figure range —or any range compatible with having hired servants.

Most working women earn less than $30,000 a year, often far less: in 1982, the average full-time employed woman earned a little over $12,000 per year. For most women, going back to work means giving up the flexibility of staying late at work, because the day-care center closes at 5:30; it means cooking dinner when you are dead tired and the baby is crabby; and it means confronting policies that maintain that you cannot take your own sick-leave time to tend a child's illness. Going back to work often leads a mother into a thicket of unsatisfactory arrangements.

Those who go back full time often feel below par for months. They usually miss their babies; something has been interrupted. As one mother said: "I don't know how other women do it. I miss her so much, and I keep calling the sitter to ask how she is."

Many women were also used to working more than forty hours a week at their jobs. But now they simply can't log in those hours without neglecting something else. Some give up sleep. One woman described how she plays with her child in the evening, then gets out her attaché case for the 9:00 P.M. to 1:00 A.M. stint. This works as long as you are strong enough to do it.

Other women find themselves working fewer hours than they used to, which sometimes causes problems on the job. In her "The Maternity Backlash" article, Anita Shreve describes how one woman came back from maternity leave to her job at an accounting firm. Before Betty had her baby, she had worked long hours. Afterward, she left at five, though others stayed late. Resentment built up, and eventually Betty left the firm. Another accountant, Elaine, who didn't have children, later expressed anger at Betty's behavior. She felt that Betty had hurt all women's chances for advancement at the firm: "Now there is a position open, and the word is out that the firm won't promote a woman to fill it. You can almost hear them saying, 'You can't expect a woman to be dedicated, because the kids come first.' "

That society does not support the working mother is a cruel reality. Without even bringing up such radical issues as government-supported day care or family allowances, we still recognize how this culture puts the working mother in such a double bind that sometimes her only choice is what lie to tell.

For example, one mother consolidated, borrowed, and used all her vacation time for the year in order to arrange eight weeks off after childbirth. (In contrast, note that most European countries require employers to pay for at least three months' maternity leave.) One morning. after she went back to work, her child looked sick.

Her day-care center has a rule against taking sick children. And her company has a policy against letting parents take sick leave when their children are sick. Should she take the child to day care and lie to the staff? Or should she call up her boss and claim that she herself is sick? Probably lying to her employer is the better course of action. At least that way she can take the child to the doctor —and hope that nobody from work sees her driving around town.

This scenario illustrates how working mothers are discouraged from taking care of their children. Somehow, even if a working mother makes a secretary's wage, she is supposed to have found the perfect mother substitute, someone available in sickness and in health—just like the women on the magazine covers. But she hasn't found a perfect mother substitute, because she can't begin to afford one. And she misses the baby while she is at work, and she has a hard time staying late. It is no wonder that many women quit after two or three months back on the job. After you have a baby, work isn't what it used to be.

Going back to work and then quitting in two months is probably the worst of the choices available. First, the mother endures full-time separation from the baby when the infant is only a few weeks old. Then, when she quits two months later, it is with a feeling of failure, a feeling of having mishandled the situation. And it all could have been prevented by arranging and timing her return to the work world in a more orderly fashion.

For all mothers, the first step to an orderly return to work is knowing your own priorities, your own goals, and your own options.

GOING BACK: YOUR GOALS AND PRIORITIES

By the time a woman is past thirty, her relationship with her baby is unlikely to be the only constraint in her life. Other areas—career, fixed expenses—look pretty immovable. What *are* your priorities and options for mothering and working?

The absolute first step in deciding about going back to work is to look into your own soul and ask yourself what you want. Despite other limiting factors, you can at least know your own mind and work toward the goal you set yourself.

For example, if you could take a six-month leave of absence but you would hate to be gone from the office that long, why do it? If your ideal of motherhood includes breastfeeding, then your choices will be very different than if your ideal of motherhood is getting good help so you won't be tied down too much.

Consider your child's needs. Babies less than six months old need nearly full-time attention from a caring adult. They are not mentally developed enough to get much out of the presence of children or toys at day care. Children of a year and a half are a different story. They may look forward to going to a place with toys and children. Part of your decision to go back to work must include your ability to obtain day care appropriate to your child's needs. The next chapter deals with this issue, and we suggest that you read it before deciding when to go back.

How much do you *care* about the job you have now? Do you see yourself as building a career that it would be very difficult to interrupt? Most women have one of two attitudes toward the work world: They see work as either an oriental bazaar or an ascending ladder.

Women who have worked at a variety of jobs may regard the whole business as a vast open-air market, where new jobs are always coming into being and old ones are always changing. A woman who has been an elementary school teacher, a secretary, and a real estate saleswoman may well hold this view. She is ready to go out there and haggle. "When I want a job," she says, "I'll have to look, but I'll find something."

On the other hand, a woman who is an accountant at a major firm may see the job market as a narrowing set of steps: "Only a few of us will make manager, and even fewer will make partner." For her, one stumble means being pushed off the ladder by the ascending hordes behind. "I've worked for years to get where I am," this woman says. "I have too much invested to jeopardize it now."

Which is your view? Does taking a few months off simply mean "How will we manage the money?" or does it also mean stepping off the ladder? And if it's the latter, is this fear realistic? It may be, but as an old and valued employee, you may have more leverage than you think, even in a competitive profession. Women have managed to become partners at law firms although they had arranged to work at reduced billing hours (part-time work) for the year after their children were born. One scientist received tenure at a prestigious government laboratory despite working part time for three years after her twin boys were born. These sorts of jobs (attempting to become a partner, getting tenure) are the ones least likely to allow for part-time work, but even here part-time work is sometimes feasible.

And what if you do fall off the ladder at your company? Ask yourself whether you need to be part of a company that has such an elaborate hierarchy and may pay relatively little. Example: An article in the *Wall Street Journal* described an advertising copywriter who quit after having a baby. The article focused on the disappointment that her boss suffered: Clients had been waiting for this copywriter to return from maternity leave before starting their ad campaigns. But the article also noted that the copywriter made $400 a week, or about $20,000 a year. A copy writer who is so good that clients wait for her can probably make far more than $20,000 a year freelance.

As one personnel officer said, "There are many people who have worked hard for their positions and therefore think that they must be making lots of money compared with other people at work. But many firms hire new people at higher salaries than they give to those promoted from within. Many long-time employees think they have golden handcuffs to the firm. Actually, the handcuffs are brass."

And how do you feel about motherhood? Consider your style of mothering from a new perspective. Every working mother must be a blend of two styles of mothering. The first style might be called "personal mothering," which includes the process of falling in love with your baby and of finding out more about yourself in an environment very different from that of the office. The second style is "executive mothering," which consists of arranging for good care for your child and not doing it all yourself.

These two styles are described as opposites, but they are truly inseparable. A complete "personal" mother could never go back to work; a complete "executive" mother would not be attuned well enough to her child to do a good job of providing for her care.

But every woman is her own mixture of these styles. What mixture are you? If you could arrange a perfect postpartum life, what would it be like? Answering some of the questions below might help.

- Your husband just inherited $20,000. Would you prefer to use this money to buy some more time off the job for yourself, or to get some live-in help so you could go back to work?

- A variation of the phantom-guarantee exercise from Chapter 6 is sometimes useful. In that chapter, we looked at phantom guarantees and their real-life equivalents as part of the "Should I have a baby?" decision. A similar exercise will help with the back-to-work decision. What guarantees would you need in order to take extra time off? A guarantee of the same job back? A promise of another job with the same company? No particular job guarantees, but the ability to borrow enough money to live on? For the moment, forget reality. This is an exercise to get you in touch with yourself and what you really want.

- Do you agree or disagree with the statement that part-time employees aren't as professional or as useful to a company as full-time employees are?

- How do you feel about women who stay home? Do you prefer to avoid them at parties, feeling that they must be leading vicarious lives through their husbands and children? Are you afraid of becoming boring? (Remember, we are not trying to tell you what women at home are really like; we're just trying to help you confront your own decision-making process. In many cases, for a working woman, part of this process is dealing with the perceived loss of status of becoming "just a housewife," however temporarily.)

Your answers to these questions will provide an indication of what you want to do, if this were the best of all possible worlds. Do you really want to take more time off, or would you rather have more help at home? How attached are you to your present position at work? At this stage, you should know what type of leave of absence you want to achieve. Now, how will you achieve it?

TO WORK OR NOT TO WORK—AND OTHER OPTIONS

Your basic options for return to work after birth:

- Take the minimum time off (two to eight weeks) and return full time.
- Take a (usually unpaid) leave of absence from your present employer (one to twelve months, or even longer).
- Return part time after the minimum time off.
- Return part time sometime later.
- Get a different part-time job, or start a business.
- Get involved in a job redefinition program (flex time, job sharing).
- Quit work and go back in a few years.
- Quit work and never go back.

Our prejudice favors the middle range of options. Going back after the minimum time is too sudden and disruptive, and quitting forever is not necessarily good for the child (unless you hate your job).

This section will therefore discuss the middle range of options (part-time work or extended leave during the first year). If you prefer to go back after the minimum time out, skip directly to Chapter 10, on choosing day care. If you are not going back to work at all, you can skip to the last chapter on guilt-free mothering.

But if you decide on part-time work or an extended leave for the first year, more questions must be answered. Unlike the first set, which involved understanding yourself, this set of questions involves assessing your external situation.

First, there is money. If you can get leave or part-time work, can you live on a smaller amount of money than you get with full-term employment? Remember, if you are taking time off you won't be paying as much for child care or new clothes for the office. But your fixed expenses, such as rent, mortgage, or car payments, are not going to change unless you do something drastic.

What is the actual dollar difference, each month, between what you need to live on and what you will have without working, or else will earn part time? Multiply this amount of money, the monthly amount, by the number of months you would like to take leave. For example, if you need $600 a month more than your husband earns in order to meet your financial obligations, and if you want to take six months' full-time leave, you will need $3,600 to do so. Do you have a source of funds you can borrow this amount of money against? Home equity, life insurance, and parents are all possible resources. Remember, we are talking about living beyond your income for only a few months to a year, not about embarking on a life of extravagance. There are times when it is reasonable to go into debt. Getting through college is one such time; beginning motherhood is another.

A word of warning: do not attempt to borrow money by living off credit cards. Unlike simple borrowing of a lump sum, credit card debt builds up insidiously, and the card companies charge outrageous interest.

While you are calculating how much money you need to borrow, also calculate how much you will actually clear if you return to work for the first months of your child's life. Day care for small infants is expensive; meals out when you are tired are expensive. Taxes are expensive, and carfare and clothes cost money. You may find that you wouldn't necessarily be earning as much as you thought. Between the cost of day care and the cost of fatigue, you are going to have to make some changes in your financial arrangements when you have a baby. Working part time for a few months is just one of the possible changes you might consider. It is not even necessarily the most expensive.

After thinking about money, it is time to think about work, and specifically about your employer.

- What are your employer's policies? As an older and probably valued employee, you may be too valuable to lose. One woman took a six-month leave of absence from a rather traditional employer. "They said they didn't want to give me an extended leave. They told me I couldn't be assured of having my old job back. I answered that I felt there would always be something useful I could do around there, and I was willing to take the chance about my old job. I knew they weren't going to get anybody who knew the company as well as I did in six months. And I was right." As several women in Chapter 3 said, "I couldn't have done this at twenty." Your age probably gives you an advantage. Try to use it. Remember, you will never get what you don't ask for.

- If your own employer is uncooperative, what about looking for temporary or less-pressured work in your own profession? Women have left cut-throat law firms for more easy-going banks; they have left research careers in medical schools for private practice, quit being private secretary to a man who never sleeps for a slot on a temporary-agency roster. Is there a way you can step down for a few years without really stepping out?

- Be realistic about working. It is nearly impossible to work at a job and take care of a baby simultaneously.

This seems obvious, but it isn't. One woman took her baby to work to nurse him. Her intentions were admirable, but her day was "a constant interruption" and her productivity was zero. Another mother decided to set up her own business in order to have time with the baby. She found herself working twelve-hour days and using day care more than if she had kept her relatively low-pressure job. On the other hand, it is possible to work from home, if you are realistic about the kind of work that you can do and how much you really need to earn to keep going. Refer to the book *Working from Home* (in the Chapter References) for more information about this.

• There are more part-time workers, freelance workers, and shared jobs now than ever before. And after all, you only need one job. Catalyst, in New York City, and New Ways to Work in San Francisco specialize in helping people arrange professional part-time situations (their addresses are in the reference section for this chapter). Even though you may not live in New York or San Francisco, you will probably find their literature and newsletters helpful. Also, in some professions (accounting, computer programming) freelancers represent a significant portion of the labor force. Your own field probably has freelancers and part-time workers. Talk to the freelancers you know. How did they arrange this for themselves? Can you do the same?

THE GRAND EXPERIMENT

Bear in mind that no mother ever feels totally reconciled to her decision. While the advantages of going back at six months instead of six weeks are clear, what is the advantage of six months over four months? What about part-time work? Is mornings-only better than three full days a week? Does it make a difference? You'll never know, because you can never tell how life would have turned out had you done things differently.

Bear in mind also that nobody is going to give you credit, as a working mother: If your child has problems, it will obviously be due to your working. If she does well, it will be despite your neglect. But at least give yourself some credit for considering your child enough to have agonized over the decision.

At a meeting recently, a mother queried Dr. Bruno Bettelheim, the well-known child psychologist: "What do you think about working mothers?" After a pause, Dr. Bettelheim replied. "I think you have asked the wrong question. The question is not, Does the mother work? The question is, How are the children being taken care of?"

Choosing
Child Care

How *are* the children being taken care of? Society as a whole hasn't got an answer to this question. It is up to you to make the best arrangements you can, and your decisions will be based on the answers you find to these questions:

- How will child care affect my child's development?
- Which child care is best for my child?
- How can I find what I want?
- How do I know if it is working well?

We would like to make universal, one-size-fits-all recommendations, but frankly, the best day care for *your* child depends on what is available. Each type varies so much in quality that what is available to you is more important than what may be best in theory.

Whichever child care you choose, the first question, "How will child care affect my child's development?" is often the most emotionally loaded one for mothers. You want to do right by your baby. You want a happy, healthy child who knows and loves you (and has not been "raised by strangers"), whose opportunities for intellectual and social development are as good as possible. Luckily, the news in this regard is quite good. Children do very well in well-chosen day care.

HOW WILL CHILD CARE AFFECT MY CHILD'S DEVELOPMENT?

The news is good, but the answers are complex. Children do very well in day care *if* the day care is a good match for the child's needs.

Let's start with the question of attachment. Psychological studies of attachment usually take the form of "strange-situation tests." In these tests, psychologists monitor the behavior of a child in the presence or absence of her mother, in a laboratory situation that is unfamiliar —strange—to the child. The researchers determine how effectively the child can use the mother as a familiar base in an unfamiliar setting. Many studies of this kind have shown that babies and toddlers who are in day care definitely prefer their mothers to the caregivers, and are as "securely attached" to their mothers as home-reared children are. Some studies have shown day-care children seeking less physical closeness to the mother in these tests, but the implications of this are unclear. A strange-situation test is, after all, a very imperfect measurement for love.

At any rate, psychological observations and testing of the children cared for part time (working hours) by competent, loving caretakers has found no evidence that such care results in psychological or emotional damage to the child. Any child placed in any type of day care before the age of one must be able to make multiple attachments and accept care from different people in order to survive, but this in itself does not seem to be detrimental.

How day care affects a child's intellectual development depends, again, on the day-care situation. Actually, considering all the varieties of day care available, we must defer anticipating what the effects are until we answer the next question: What types of care are best?

WHAT CHILD CARE IS BEST FOR MY CHILD?

Unfortunately, psychological research is not very helpful at answering this question, because it has only recently begun to address the tremendous variations found in day-care situations. We will quote research here, but ultimately we have to depend on common sense.

What have psychologists studied? At first, they studied orphanages and foundling homes. These understaffed places, right out of Dickens, were so bad that many of the babies placed in them simply did not survive. Predictably, the results of these studies showed that "day care" was terrible for babies.

After a while, foundling homes disappeared, so psychologists began to study better day-care centers. As a matter of fact, since the investigators were often faculty members, they tended to do their research at well-run, model facilities connected with the university's child development department. This answered the question "What effect does a large, well-run day-care center have on the development of faculty children?"

Psychologists are just beginning to ask other essential questions: What effect does in-home day care have on a child? What effect does family day care have on a child? How do large day-care centers differ? How does the personality of the child matter in all of this? The answers are not yet fully available. Half the children in America are participating in a grand experiment. But today's mothers can't wait for thirty years to find out the results that will tell them what to do; they have to make decisions now.

Some things *are* known about day care and child development, and these facts can help you pick the best situation for your child. Before we go further with advice, though, we need to define our terms: What is in-home child care, family day care, or a day-care center? What are the pros and cons of each of these arrangements? What are your options?

The Child-Care Thicket

In-home Day Care

This is care for the child in your own home. In this case, the caretaker may be a relative. If the child's father is available, he is the prime candidate. Other possibilities include grandparents and aunts of the child (your parents or siblings or in-laws). A caretaker who is a member of the family has many advantages; relatives really care about the child. Also, arrangements with relatives tend to be more stable than other arrangements. Housekeepers may come and go, but grandmothers tend to stay awhile.

Some studies indicate that over half of the children of working mothers are cared for by relatives. Perhaps the reports of the death of the extended family are exaggerated.

Another option for in-home care is hiring a person who is not related to you. The quality of this care depends almost completely on the personality of the woman (or more rarely, man) you hire. She may be a high-priced nanny, an illegal alien, a recent high-school graduate, or an older retired woman. The most important question is, How well does she take care of your child?

The major advantage of in-home care is that the child stays in her own surroundings, and so the mother usually has a great deal of control over how her child is cared for. The disadvantages are two: expense and impermanence.

Child care in your home will usually cost more than the minimum wage per hour. It also embroils the parents in a very dense thicket of government regulations. You must pay a social security tax if you employ someone, even part time. Then there are state and federal tax withholding, unemployment compensation tax, and other drains on the family budget and patience. And of course, don't forget penalties for filling out the government paperwork incorrectly.

Of course, some employees may prefer to be paid under the table, so that they don't have to declare this income. Illegal aliens and women on welfare often fit this classification. How you feel about these less-formal pay arrangements is between you and your local law enforcement agency. You might also remember that if the employee isn't bringing your money to the attention of the IRS, you probably can't deduct the money from your income taxes, either. Losing your child-care deduction is a direct loss to your pocketbook, not even counting the legal problems that might ensue if you are caught.

Another problem is uncertainty about how long the worker will stay. Some people are lucky, and hire women who remain with the family for years and years. Most people are not so fortunate. A teen-age girl may decide to go to college after a few months; an older woman may decide the work is too demanding as soon as the baby starts to crawl. If you were only planning to use child care in your home for a few months or a year (which is what we recommend), this may not be a problem. If you are planning home care for several years, you will probably have a series of caretakers over that period of time.

Family Day Care

This is care for your children at another woman's home. There are three things to consider in choosing a family-care home: the personality and competence of the woman running the home; the physical home environment; and how many other children are being taken care of at the same time.

Family day-care homes can be splendid, or they can be places where an overworked woman tries to oversee too many children without much of a break. (We believe that more than three children under two years old is too many.) Is the house cheerful, and do the children seem content when you drop in unexpectedly? Or is the TV the prime baby-sitter? A day-care home can provide an excellent family-style setting, which is stimulating and supportive to a young child, or it can be a dreary place to "park" a child until the end of the day.

Day-Care Centers

These are specially set up environments other than homes where twenty-five to several hundred children are cared for at a time. The facilities range from church social halls to buildings devoted entirely to child care. Again, the quality of the care varies greatly. The average enrollment in these centers is growing from forty to eighty children, in an effort to offset rising costs. The staff-child ration varies—from one adult to each of four infants, five toddlers, or eight preschoolers to whatever the traffic will bear or is required by law.

The advantage of a big place is the availability of many toys, activities, and playmates. The disadvantages include possible spread of disease, overcrowding, and often inadequate staff with high job turnover. Day-care centers often pay very low wages for very demanding work. Staff turnover is less upsetting to the older child, who focuses on his playmates, than it is to the young child, who needs a lot of consistent interaction with his caretaker.

We tend to agree with Bryna Siegal-Gorelick, in *The Working Parents' Guide to Child Care,* when she notes that "I have never seen a franchised infant or toddler program that I felt was really good. . . . As far as I'm concerned, it's not possible to provide good quality care for children under three and still make a corporation-sized profit. . . . There are, however, many good run-for-profit programs for children three years and older."

Not all day-care centers are run for profit, however. The ones subsidized by corporations tend to be well staffed, with low child-teacher ratios and a great deal of parent involvement in the center. For example, Syntex, a large pharmaceutical company in Palo Alto, California, has company-subsidized care for the children of employees at its own center near corporate headquarters. The children appreciate knowing that they are at the day-care center connected with Mommy's or Daddy's work. They also enjoy the center's frequent field trips to Syntex.

We do not mean to imply that all large centers are ghastly places.

In any case, the advantages of large day-care centers are chiefly applicable to older children. Toys, other children, field trips, and structured activities are exciting to the three-year-old, and basically irrelevant to the six-month-old. And so it seems that we cannot even give straightforward advantages and disadvantages to the various types of day care without considering the age and development of the child.

Day Care Through the Ages: From Infancy to Childhood

The Developing Infant

Babies grow at a phenomenal rate, not only physically but emotionally, intellectually, and socially. A caring mother who can't be there herself is concerned about her child's growth in all of these areas. But let us start with the basics. At the end of a day, you mainly want for a six-week-old to be fed, content, and healthy. Developmental matters are important, but step one is simply keeping the baby's physical development unimpaired by poor nutrition or disease.

This can be trickier than it might seem. Because when day care is started with babies this young, a number of special issues arise.

The first concerns breast feeding, and the determined mother who says, "I can return to work full time when the baby is six weeks old and continue to breastfeed." We hate to be so negative on a subject we are so positive about, but this is nearly impossible to do.

If you plan to fully nurse your baby but can nurse her only in the morning, at lunch break, and again after work, you are being completely unrealistic. Small babies simply eat more often than that. And if you encourage the caregiver to give bottles, the bottles will quickly replace your breast, since it is difficult for a very young baby to learn two styles of sucking (bottle and breast).

If you really want to nurse your baby, it is best to wait three months or so before going back to work full time. After three months, the baby is much more likely to learn two styles of sucking. Then the mother can provide bottles for the time she is away at work, and the baby can still be nursed as long as mother and baby both want. After four months, the baby can be fed solids in the mother's absence. Just a few weeks makes a tremendous difference!

If you do decide to go back full time at six weeks, however, face the fact that this by default constitutes a decision to wean the baby from the breast, and make sure that your child-care arrangements include protecting the baby from disease. Expressing milk is fine for an occasional relief bottle, but it is usually impractical for full-time nourishment of a baby.

Which brings us to the next issue: Babies are not, immunologically, the same as adults. The antibodies in breast milk provide a good deal of protection from infection. If the baby is no longer nursing, you must be very careful not to increase his exposure to disease at the same time.

Unfortunately, uninformed mothers risk their baby's health when they discontinue nursing and return to full-time work. They take the baby off breast milk and simultaneously take him from the confined circle of home; then he is put in a large day-care center, with many children coming and going. The results are predictable. The baby gets sick.

In an informal sample of mothers and doctors, we found that many babies end up taking antibiotics within four weeks of arriving in day care. The major problems are ear infections and diarrhea. Many diseases that are merely inconvenient for an older child can be actively dangerous for a baby, especially diarrhea-type disorders.

This sickness is to be expected. All over the world, the newly weaned child is the one most vulnerable to disease. Medical anthropologists have a name for the set of problems that attack (and often kill) third-world children:

"weanling diarrhea." These children die because they have inadequate nutrition, lose the antibody protection of breast milk, and begin drinking the contaminated local water supply, all at the same time.

It is not our intention to be alarmist, and certainly, conditions in the United States are not nearly that bad: Bottles, clean water, and good medical care are readily available. Your baby will not die of day care. Nevertheless, it is wise to minimize your child's exposure to diseases, which are especially prevalent in large day-care centers.

Hepatitis is one example. Dr. Stephan Handler, chief epidemiologist for hepatitis at the Center for Disease Control in Atlanta, was quoted in the *Wall Street Journal* about hepatitis outbreaks in day-care centers. Phoenix, Arizona, in 1978 and 1979, had its share of such an epidemic when 20 percent of all centers with diapered children had hepatitis outbreaks. Handler estimates that 15 percent of infectious hepatitis cases in this country are acquired through day-care facilities. This 15 percent estimate includes adult hepatitis: Parents catch it from their children.

In another case, the Center for Disease Control in Atlanta studied a facility in that city where more than half of the toddlers were infected with the parasite *giardia lamblia,* which causes diarrhea. The rate of parasite infection for children cared for at home was less than 2 percent. According to Dr. Bartlett of the University of Texas, placing a child in a day-care setting increases her chance of getting diarrhea by least 30 percent. As mentioned before, diarrhea can be much more dangerous for a baby or toddler (who loses a high percentage of body fluids rather quickly) than it is for an adult.

As a general rule, there is more disease in bigger centers. As Dr. Handler says, "The larger the center or the longer the hours, the greater the chance [of disease]."

And then there are drop-ins. It is the policy of most for-profit day-care centers to accept drop-in children, who are not regularly enrolled. Molly McCarthy, vice-president of La Petite Academy, explains in the *Wall Street Journal* that the shorter the time the child is cared for, the more profitable the child is to the center. The problem is that drop-ins are often ill children who have been excluded from their regular center.

We recommend that you avoid weaning the child from breast milk when you place her in day care, and that you choose a day-care center small enough to minimize the baby's exposure to disease from other children. Care in your own home is ideal. If that cannot be arranged, care in a family day-care center (someone else's home), where the person cares for the minimum number of children (preferably just hers and yours), is the next best.

So now, with nutrition and health acknowledged, it is time to remember that a baby is more than a body. He is also a total learning system. The caregiver is the teacher in a beginning course in life. The infant has to find out who he is, in the most elemental way, whom he can trust, and what he can do. His early experiences are the basis for his later learning and for his trust in the world. Are his caretakers reliable? Can he learn to expect what happens next?

The very first milestones in a baby's life seem to be built in. With adequate care, the baby will start to smile at two months. With a reasonable amount of attention, she will discover her feet and play with her toes. Even as early as six months, however, a baby's perceptive and cognitive skills are related to the quality of interaction she has had with a nurturing caretaker. Infants need a lot of attention.

They need the attention because, after about six to eight months, the milestones become more complex and more dependent on the environment the infant has had. The baby is discovering cause-and-effect relationships and is beginning to learn language, at least in a passive manner. At this point, the baby's social environment begins to have a very noticeable effect on his development. Do people talk to him a lot? If he is a jumpy baby, have people learned how to calm him down? If he is a quiet baby, do people take the time to stimulate him or do they just say, "Thank heavens, he's easy," and ignore him? It is clear that the quality of his care at six months also depends on whether your baby's caretaker got to know his individual patterns at earlier stages in his development. Therefore, it is best if the child has the same caretaker for the first year of his life, either in your home or in a family day-care home with very few children.

The six-month-old is not developmentally equipped to get much out of the presence of other children. She is busy discovering herself and the world around her. Social interaction with peers really comes much later. A caretaker who wheels her for a walk in the stroller, pointing out the birds and trees, or who chats gently with her as she makes lunch is doing the right thing for her cognitive development. Lying in a crib with a mobile or even playing with "educational" toys is no substitute for the personal attention of a caring adult.

The Older Baby (One to Two Years Old)

The one-year-old can often say a few words and walk. If he cannot do so at one, he will learn rather quickly within the next few months. At this age a baby is really interested in other children, other toys, and other sights. Family day care is usually preferable now to day care in your home.

The beginnings of friendship come now. If your child has another near his own age to play with, the two may well become baby friends. While earlier theories of child-rearing implied that social play was developmentally possible only for the child over three years old, more recent work has shown that a year-old toddler can begin to have "one good friend." Play between two children is usually more satisfying and intellectually worthwhile than is play with many children, at least at this age.

While peer interaction helps even a very young (around one year old) child's social skills, more peers are not necessarily better. Bigger can even be worse. A child psychologist, who did not want her name used because she still does research at day-care centers, noted that she has a hard time getting research accomplished in large centers. The child-to-staff ratio at these centers is often high, and any adult who enters is quickly surrounded by children who need some help or who are crying, but cannot get anyone on the staff to pay attention. She can't get her research done, and she also notes that it is difficult for the children to learn anything of value while they are crying.

A one-year-old is still a very small child. He isn't toilet trained; somebody has to change his diapers. He has a "remarkable curiosity," as Dr. Burton White says. This curiosity, coupled with his ability to move around at will, is certain to get him into danger if he is not watched carefully.

Moreover, his language development is now at a crucial phase. For good language development, a child between one and two needs frequent interactions with an adult or much older child. Alison Clarke-Stewart, of the University of Chicago, in her book *Daycare*, notes the differences between mothers and teachers in this regard. Conversations between child and teacher tend to be much shorter than conversations between a child and her mother. Conversations with the teacher are also more likely to be initiated by the teacher for a specific purpose, and are less likely to be initiated by the child.

Home day-care mothers seem to fall midway between mothers and teachers in terms of language. They are more likely to talk on a one-to-one basis with children, and they are often more sensitive to the individual interests, needs, and communication styles of the child. On the minus side, they are cooler and more emotionally aloof, less playful and stimulating than mothers.

We do recommend family day care for a child this age, rather than a large center, so when you choose a family day-care home, try to choose one with a mother who will chat with your child, and who perhaps has another child near your child's age for her to play with.

The Preschool Child (Two to Three Years Old and Older)

When your child is around the age of three, the good day-care center comes into its own. Three-year-olds are toilet-trained and verbal. They interact well with other children. It is at this stage that children in day care often do better on standardized tests than home-reared children do. As Clarke-Stewart notes, day-care children "do better in tests of verbal fluency, memory, and comprehension. . . . Their speech is more complex, and they are able to identify other people's feelings and points of view earlier. . . . Daycare teaches children things they wouldn't have learned at home . . . concepts, arithmetic." Day care seems to be most intellectually advantageous for children from poorer families, but children from more affluent homes also benefit.

Even if a mother does not choose to work when her child is this age, she may want to put him into a good nursery school every morning, just to give some of the benefits of day care!

The concerns about disease also diminish for three-year-olds. Diapered children are the ones most likely to spread and get hepatitis and diarrhea. Older children in day care tend to get more colds than do home-reared children, but the intellectual advantages offset this disadvantage. All in all, it is the lucky child who is in good day care or nursery school at three.

In choosing child care, try to select the type that will best benefit your child's developmental age. We recommend mother care at home for the young infant; home or a small family-care home for the older baby; and a larger, well-run center for the preschool child.

And remember, children develop at different rates. A recommendation to send a three-year-old to center day care presumes that he is a reasonably well-developed three-year-old. Some children (boys especially) develop their language ability slowly. Such a child can often benefit a longer period of time with extra attention in family day care.

Once you have decided on the type of day care you want, the next problem is finding it.

HOW CAN I FIND GOOD DAY CARE?

Day care is easy to find. Just consult any metropolitan-area phone book, and you will see large display ads for the franchised centers and smaller ads for local centers. When your child is three years old, the best day care can be found in the Yellow Pages.

When your child is an infant, however, this is not the case. As noted above, the best day care for an infant is in your own home or in a family day-care home. The people providing this kind of care do not advertise in the phone books, and the good ones can be hard to find.

Local resources in your community may be able to help you. For example, Bananas, a child-care information resource service in Oakland, California, has established a successful model program, and IBM is developing a national referral network to benefit employees. Your pediatrician should know of the child-care resources and referral services in your community.

But according to the mothers we talked to, word of mouth seems to be the best way of finding day care for an infant. Talk to people while you are pregnant, tell them what you want, ask them if they know somebody. If you choose to put up an ad, the bulletin boards of a senior citizens center or a college might be the right place. Do you know anyone acquainted with people who have just immigrated to this country? One of the happiest babies we know is routinely cared for by an older Russian Jewish woman who came to this country three years ago. Her English is spotty but her heart is warm, and she really understands babies. Another well-cared-for baby was loved through the first year of her life by an illegal immigrant from Mexico.

Which brings up, once again, the subject of legality. We do not encourage you to break any laws. But there is a problem in this world: Child-care employment doesn't usually pay enough to people who need a middle-class type of income. So we must tell you that many otherwise law-abiding women are making legally questionable arrangements for child care. And while every state has a day-care home licensing procedure, many excellent family day-care homes are unlicensed. As Seigal-Gorelick says in her book *Working Parents' Guide to Child Care:* "Licensing is no assurance of the quality of care! . . . Among day-care mothers I've known, I'd guess that only 10 percent have been licensed." We are not advocating that you do anything illegal; we are just telling you the state of things in the real world.

When it comes to choosing a woman to work in your home, or finding one who runs a family day-care center, the personality of the woman should be the first consideration. Look for someone trustworthy, kind, competent, and reliable. If at all possible, get recommendations from other women she has worked for. If you can spend a fair amount of money, you might want to hire a woman from the special agencies providing trained nannies.

But don't choose a woman just because she comes from an agency of some sort. Some "agencies" will hire anyone who needs a few dollars and seems sober at the time. Nobody but you can really decide whether this is the person to take care of your child. That decision is your responsibility.

For a family day-care home, look for one that has a kind, competent person, a reasonable amount of space and toys, and not too many children. When it comes to number of children, remember that many family day-care mothers have several children coming after school, as well as the children cared for during the day. This may result in a two-hour period each day when there are too many children for the woman to handle. Family day-care homes are often licensed for more children per caretaker than large centers are. If the woman is overloaded with children, and if there is a steady stream of new children coming into the home, a family day-care home loses all its advantages over center care for the young child.

The best family day-care woman is usually a mother earning some money while her own children are small. She should be someone you can talk to, someone who will be open with you about how your child is doing and point out any problems that you might want to address. (This is true for any child-care person you hire.)

Just because a woman has been doing family day-care for a long time is not really a recommendation. The day-care mother is home all day with several small children; she is tied down. After a few years, burnout becomes a very real issue. The children begin to all look the same; she may begin to see them as difficult and ungrateful.

For an older child (three and up), choices are easier. You want an environment that is stimulating but safe. The exact personality of the caretaker is not as big an issue, and rules are easier to formulate. There should be some organized teaching programs and some free play. Parental involvement in running the center (a parents' board, parent volunteer days for jungle-gym building or field trips) is a good sign. The outdoor play areas should be easily accessible. The child-staff ratio should be sufficient to prevent neglect and to protect the weaker or less assertive children. A one-to-twelve ratio is legal in many states, but we recommend a one-to-nine ratio.

Visit several centers. Spend at least an hour in each one. How do the children behave? Are they happy or whiny? (Crying, fighting children are a sign of understaffing.) Are the toys in use, are the children comfortable? While you can almost certainly decide for yourself whether this is a place in which your child will be happy, some of the references in this book's bibliography section can give more specific guidelines about finding good day-care centers.

Once you have chosen a good day-care home or a good day-care provider, you've taken care of 90 percent of your day-care needs. But not all of the needs.

Backups Are Essential

In order to work reliably at your job, you will need two kinds of backup day care: one for when the child is sick, and one for when the day-care provider (be she someone who comes to your home or the mother in the family day-care home) is sick. You cannot afford to miss work whenever one or the other happens. (We are talking about relatively minor illnesses here, not hospitalization.) If you have one day-care provider in your home, you must count on the fact that sometimes she will get sick or need a vacation. And if you have family or center day-care, they may refuse to take your sick child.

Perhaps you have a relative or friend who is willing to do occasional duty. Work out tentative arrangements in advance, not at 7:30 A.M. the day of the emergency. Perhaps this is where the local agencies that provide practical nurses can be of help. At any rate, decide what you are going to do *before* the dread morning arrives. Some communities have warm lines or hot lines for care of sick children. Simply staying home from work whenever your child or your sitter is mildly ill is usually the least acceptable of the alternatives.

HOW CAN I TELL IF IT IS WORKING WELL?

Once you have chosen your day care, the next step is making sure that it is working well, both for you and your child. The first way to do this is to check it out yourself. Drop in at the center, the family day-care home, or your own home (if you have in-home help). Stop in unexpectedly, at three in the afternoon or ten in the morning. Obviously, you can't do this every day, but you can do it occasionally. How are things going?

One of the troubles with day care is that infants and small children can't give you a decent report of what is going on. A fourth grader will tell you exactly what a "mean" thing his teacher did, but an infant will tell you nothing. The responsibility is yours.

Perhaps you think that all this warning is theoretical. We assure you, it is not. There are some fine day-care homes and centers in this world, and there are others that count on the fact that babies are not squealers.

Some large centers have policies against parents visiting unexpectedly or to observe. ("Visits confuse the children and disrupt their day.") Parents coming to pick up their children stay in a separate waiting room while the children's names are called by loudspeaker. The parents are not encouraged to see where the children spend the day, or to talk to the staff about their child's progress.

The above description is not a horror story, but a description of a large day-care center within four miles of one of our homes. There are no reports of child abuse from this center or any "real" evidence that anything is wrong there. Nevertheless, we would not recommend that you take your child to such a place. We believe that parents should have more knowledge—and more control—than a center like this is willing to provide.

Even if you have chosen a good day-care situation for your child, children and day-care situations can both change over time. Sometimes you have to switch in order to continue to get good care for your child. But of course you don't want to move your child around too often.

How to Tell When It Is Time to Change

If your ten-month-old daughter or year-old son suddenly starts crying and grabbing for you when you leave him at the center, don't panic. This is simply called separation anxiety. Babies get it right on schedule in the second half of the first year, and then get over it around the beginning of the second year. A milder form of separation anxiety often strikes between the ages of two and a half and three. In neither case is it the fault of the day-care center, nor do the tears mean the child will be unhappy all day.

On the other hand, if your child seems out of sorts or depressed (yes, young children can get depressed), or if the day-care mother or staff don't seem to be as open with you as they used to be, things may not be going well. Sometimes, at a big center, several staff leave at once, as if resigning were contagious. Under these circumstances, begin dropping in at odd times: See how things are going. Your child's caretakers may be overloaded or burnt out. It may be time for a change.

You have to know your own child. How is he or she reacting to the experience of day care? Is his language development within the norms for his age? Is he friendly and outgoing, or does he tend to pick fights with other children? You must keep in touch. Keeping in touch will prevent the major disasters (sexual abuse of children) and the more minor misfortunes (having a child cared for by a burnt-out, crabby staff member). When in doubt, drop in.

Why don't parents drop in more often at their child's day-care centers? Of course, the parents work, and their jobs are demanding. But sometimes parents don't drop in because of guilt. They regret having the child in day care, and so they don't want to look: If they close their eyes those eight hours of the child's life will go away. Is this guilt necessary? Is it even helpful?

WILL I BE A "BAD" MOTHER IF I LEAVE MY CHILD?

The mother who hates to be home is unlikely to be truly loving to her child. On the other hand, a mother who hates to leave her child is rather likely to have a child who adjusts poorly to day care: "If Mommy thinks that leaving me here is so awful, I can't possibly be happy here."

It seems reasonable that the children of happy working mothers left in the care of competent caretakers would be better off than being with an unhappy mother who stays home. Research in this area is mixed and sometimes difficult to interpret. Nevertheless, it does suggest that daughters of working mothers tend to have higher career goals, more self-esteem, and do better in school. Children of working mothers also have less rigid ideas of how roles and activities are differentiated by sex. They see more similarities in what men and women do (they both work, they both take care of children and do household tasks) than the children of nonworking mothers.

Older children, especially, benefit from the increased household responsibilities that they usually have when both parents are working. This presumes, of course, that the parents don't feel so guilty about working that they arrange for their children to have everything but do nothing. Having an adult woman as a full-time servant is not actually good for an older child's development.

Working mothers are also healthier and less likely to be depressed than nonworking mothers. This may come from the enhanced sense of self that is the result of fulfilling several roles successfully, or from having more adult contacts, or simply from having more money.

We recommend that mothers stay home with six-week-olds. However, once your children are no longer babies, it is usually better to find good child care and go back to work, if that is what you are inclined to do. With good child care, you can be a happy, healthy working mother, with self-esteem and even money, and have bright, happy, and responsible children.

THE OLDER BUT WISER MOTHER: AN EXPERIENCED CHOOSER

As we noted in Chapter 1 of this book, the older mother has several advantages. She is usually more attuned to her baby, and she is often more financially secure. In choosing day care, her insight into what the child needs, as well as the financial resources available to her, definitely serve her well. But she has other advantages. She knows her own mind, and she knows quality. The older mother is not easily bamboozled into accepting shoddy goods, or poor-quality care. She has also had extensive experience with people. Compared with the average twenty-year-old, the woman of thirty is far more adept at predicting how people will behave in various circumstances. This helps her immensely in hacking her way through the child-care thicket, and especially in the intensely personal and individualistic task of choosing day care for a baby.

Moreover, she is in touch with her own baby, and knowing a child's needs and knowing how to provide for them is the essence of choosing day care. Actually, this is the essence of many of the tasks of motherhood. Working mother or homebody mother, some things never change. The good mother will take the time to arrange for good day care, just as she takes the time to play with her baby.

Beyond Guilt

We're not going to tell you that you shouldn't feel guilty (although there is nothing to feel guilty about). We don't want to add yet another layer of guilt: "I feel guilty, but I know I shouldn't."

Instead, we would like to explore what there is about modern motherhood that is so guilt-provoking, and offer some ideas for a life with some inner serenity. But for modern women, the first stage in achieving serenity is examining guilt.

Why is motherhood so difficult nowadays? The '80s are, in many ways, the best decade women have ever lived in. Reproductive choice is possible, decent jobs are possible. Sexual discrimination still exists, but it is not as blatant and overt as it was twenty years ago. In most ways, life for women is better than it was twenty, or even ten, years ago.

So why is there so much unhappiness? Why do intelligent women who choose to have children have so many problems with guilt?

UNREALISTIC EXPECTATIONS: THE ROAD TO GUILT IS PAVED WITH GOOD INTENTIONS

Guilt is not an automatic part of motherhood; it is a direct consequence of unrealistic expectations. For example, 100 years ago, mothers could not realistically expect that all their children would live to adulthood. Therefore, there is no evidence in the literature of those times that mothers felt guilty, or that anybody particularly blamed them, when children died young. Mothers had sorrow, but there is no evidence that they had overwhelming bouts of guilt.

Often there wasn't even that much sorrow, especially in poor families, or if the children died as babies. "He's well settled" (in heaven), poor mothers would say after the death of a child. Considering that the child might well have gone to bed hungry most nights, being settled in heaven may have looked very good. Back on earth, there was also one less mouth to feed and often another baby on the way.

What about feeling guilty about how the children turned out? Such guilt used to be the exception, rather than the rule. Of course, some children really disgraced the family, but that was rare. And the parents were more often pitied than blamed, even in these circumstances.

What about children who didn't do well in school? A modern mother might well feel guilty: Perhaps she should not have gone back to work. Perhaps she should not have had another child so quickly. Should she have done or not done any number of things?

For most mothers 100 years ago, such questions would not have even been asked. In England, for example, except for the wealthy, children started working by the time they were twelve. Boys worked in the fields or mines, or else were apprenticed out. Girls were sent to live in other homes, "in service," doing housework for pay and visiting their own homes only on holiday. If the children were moral (and at age twelve, most are) when they began their working lives, and if they were reasonably hard workers, it was assumed that their parents had raised them well. Raising a child to be moral and a hard worker at twelve was within the realm of possibility for most children and most mothers.

Well, times have changed, and in many ways for the better: Children have a greater chance of survival now, and will not be sent out to work at age twelve. On the other hand, the expectations mothers now have about their children have swelled to often unrealistic proportions. It is a lot harder to raise a superstar child, who gets A's in every facet of his extended schooling and copes well with an affluent adolescence, than it is to raise a child who is a good worker at twelve. Not all children will win scholarships to Harvard, no matter what you do as a mother.

The basis for this modern guilt is a belief in the perfectability of children by means of perfect mothering, especially by perfect mothering in the first years of life. This belief is carried to extremes in what Jonathan Kirsch called the "gourmet baby" phenomenon, in a witty article published in *California* magazine.

In this article, Kirsch describes mothers who are "not afraid" of the "genius syndrome." They are using flash cards, called "bits," to teach their one-year-olds to identify Beethoven and Bach, the parts of a piano, First Ladies, the anatomy of a horse—and, of course, to read. Younger babies are taught to swim, taken to workout classes, massaged. As Kirsch describes it, "Infancy [is considered] a window of opportunity: the first baby step down the long road to self-perfection. . . . [The parents believe that] the better baby will grow up to be a better adult."

As Kirsch notes, the old-fashioned indulged baby had it easier. She was gifted with an "imported pram, and English nanny, a pony. In return, the blue-blooded baby [was] expected only to show some breeding and refrain from wetting the oriental carpet." The gourmet baby, on the other hand, is considered to be perfectable, through the strenuous efforts of her mother.

Of course, not all mothers begin working on the perfectability of their babies in this way. But though most mothers believe that ten months is too early to start using flash cards, they still think that the child is simply a product of how good a job the mother did. And the stakes are very high.

Let us look at this belief for a moment. It is very pervasive but extremely destructive of good mother-child relationships. For one thing, there are no perfect children, any more than there are perfect adults.

The Myth of the Perfect Mother

Beginning with Freud and continuing with John Bowlby's *Love and Attachment,* published in 1951, the mother's absence or inadequate caretaking has been blamed for all the ills that flesh is heir to. If the mother had only done a good job of mothering, her child would never get into fights, do badly in math, goof off at violin lessons, or behave in any other inconvenient way.

Bowlby's monographs have had an extraordinary effect on the world of child-rearing. They are echoed to this day in recent books such as *Creative Parenting,* by William Sears. Actually, Bowlby did not even study children who lived with their mothers when he wrote his books. He drew his conclusions about the necessity for a "warm, intimate, and continuous relationship with [the] mother" while studying children who were orphaned or separated from their families by World War II. These children were living in institutions.

It was clear to Bowlby that these institutionalized children needed mothers. They probably did. From there he went on to emphasize the necessity for "continuity" of the relationship between mother and child. "Such enjoyment and close indication of feeling is only possible if the relationship is continuous. Much emphasis has already been laid on the necessity of continuity for the growth of the child's personality."

Continuity of care soon began to mean that the mother should never leave the baby. More recently, another male expert, Dr. William Sears, explains why the mother must be there: "Why is substitute care-giving second best? The substitute mother may not be able to pick up on the baby's cues and sense what he needs. . . . In addition to these needs, babies also have their stress periods which cannot be scheduled for weekends or after working hours. Only you can effectively parent your baby through these stress periods because only you can be perfectly attuned to his needs."

In this way, a mother might, if she works, miss out on being around for a stress period (crabby period? colicky period?). And that, apparently, would be terrible for the baby, who would lose self-esteem in the process, since, according to Sears, "Babies learn resignation easily. They learn to accept unfulfilled needs, but at the price of lowered self-esteem and trust in their environment."

The implication of Bowlby's and Sears's work, is that if a child has a truly full-time, perfect mother who makes sure to be present at all the periods of fussiness or whininess and who is completely attuned, that child will grow up to be perfect. In other words, if a mother has to go away, or else needs a break or some income and can't be in two places at once, she will have an imperfect child and will *deserve* to feel guilty.

Bowlby and Sears aren't the only ones looking for perfect mothers, however. Psychiatric literature is full of mothers who didn't make it to perfection. A recent article, "Mother-Blaming in Major Clinical Journals," by Caplan and Hall-McCorquodale, pointed out: "The child's pathology was attributed at least in part to the mother's activity in 82 percent of the articles. . . . Thus, the mother's activity was regarded as harmful more than four-fifths of the time. . . ."

In short, maintaining that mothers shouldn't feel guilty about their inability to be perfect becomes a downright radical statement. Blaming the mother is an old indoor sport in the mental health profession. Bowlby and Sears point out that the mother might leave, and the psychiatrists suspect that she might do something wrong. And the sport is not restricted to professionals. Even common speech blames the mother. As Letty Pogrebin notes, a bad woman is a bitch, but a bad man is a "son of a bitch" or a "bastard," both of which terms implicate his mother.

If the goal is perfect children through perfect mothering, it is no wonder that most flesh-and-blood mothers fail. A mother might actually want a break from her child's stress period, and she wouldn't mind if the baby learned a little resignation. She might not want to be 100-percent responsible for twenty-four-hour coverage. Some of her actions might turn out to be detrimental to the child. She might be human, instead of perfect.

The modern mother, surrounded by such falls from grace, is a long way from the women who thought well of themselves if their children were decent workers at the age of twelve.

And they not only have to strive for perfect motherhood, they are also urged and expected to continue climbing the corporate ladder to a successful career.

THE CATCH-22 OF MOTHERHOOD

The debate with no final answer goes on: Where should you be, at work or at home?

Of course, even if you stay home full-time for the child's entire life, you are not guaranteed a perfect product, for all your effort at polishing and buffing, because children, as you well know, are not products. They are themselves, people you are raising.

But you are a person, too, and it is not necessarily true that staying home full time will make you the best mother for your child. One woman who gave up a fifteen-hour-a-day career as a vice-president of a growing corporation to stay home with her child commented, "I used to be obsessive about my career; now I'm obsessive about my child." Her child has just turned one, and she worries about becoming rather too controlling a mother, now that the rigors of the first few months are over. This woman's personal development goals should probably include an attempt at balance. Unfortunately, society will not support her in that choice. Society as a whole understands working fifteen hours a day at a job or being a full-time mother. It doesn't understand the concept of a balanced life very well at all.

Society's lack of support is really the catch-22 of mothering. A great deal of lip service is paid to staying home with the child, but very little attention gets paid to how to help mothers stay home for a while without dropping out of the human race. Mothers and babies are cooped up together, in their separate and segregated homes. And being at home with a small child can be lonely. "I miss the people at the office, the interaction, the chatting," said the mother quoted above. "It used to be my social life, as well as my job. I take my daughter to a baby gym program, and I talk to the mothers there for a while, but it is not the same. I'm only there about two hours a week, and we are supposed to be 'with the kids,' not talking to each other, anyway. It's not like the office."

Only in the Western world is taking on the task of motherhood so isolating. In other cultures, women work more in groups. They go out to the fields in groups, carrying their hoes and their nursing babies. They associate with each other in ways that are directly related to their daily, productive work. And there is usually someone else around to watch the child for a few minutes.

Going to the bathroom is more of a crisis for an American mother of a crawling baby than it is for an African or Fijian mother. The American mother must calculate: "If I put him in his playpen suddenly, he may cry. If I leave him out, he may pull over the lamp. But I only have to urinate, so maybe this time I can let him crawl around." She must plan to spend her time in the bathroom either listening to his howls or keeping her ears open for the sound of the lamp tipping over. The African mother simply asks another mother to watch the child a few minutes. She will certainly do the same for the other mother's child. In child-rearing, many hands not only make light the work, they make the work possible, while adult companionship makes it pleasant.

Motherhood as a Career

> There is no single job in America more economically perilous today than that of full-time motherhood. . . . Any woman selfish enough to want to take care of her own children had better find a husband who will never leave her and never get sick . . . and never, ever, die.
>
> —Ellen Goodman,
> Pulitzer Prize–winning columnist,
> in her book *At Large*

Motherhood is a terrible career. Not only are the working conditions difficult, the job security is awful. Nearly half of all marriages end in divorce. Even if a woman stays married, husbands tend to be older than their wives and their life-spans shorter, so the average married woman has widowhood in her future. If she is unlucky enough, she may well be putting a child through college during that widowhood. Simple economics indicates that a resumé with only the word *mother* on it is a very bad idea.

Few women who have had children in their thirties have or want such a resumé. They plan to return to full-time work, maybe after a year or perhaps not for a few years. But as Goodman says, the women with the "greatest sense of choice about mothering are those few who have been told the door to the office will still be open. Only they can look at mothering as 'time out' rather than a permanent job disability."

Unfortunately, devoting yourself to motherhood for a few months can often feel like walking the gangplank of a ship, stepping off into a world of isolation from other adults and perhaps watching the office door slam shut behind you. And as it shuts, your ability to financially survive divorce or widowhood shuts also. Again, this is society's trap, not something intrinsic to motherhood. During wars, men leave for the front and the government makes laws (veterans' preferences) to make it easy for them to be hired when they come back. Motherhood, however, is not as vital to national interests as armies are, and so it is probably too much to expect that we'll ever see the equivalent of a G.I. Bill for motherhood.

We would disagree with Goodman in one regard, however. She describes the few who "have been told" that the door to the office will still be open. We do not recommend that a woman of thirty wait around to be "told" that there will still be jobs similar to hers after she takes time off for motherhood. If the woman needs to be told by somebody, we will be happy to do so: Offices will still be there four months or three years from now. It would be nice if your boss held your job for you; it would be convenient, it would even be flattering. But it is not a necessity for beginning the adventure of motherhood.

Because what it comes down to is that, as a woman entering motherhood, you must set your own priorities. Society, with its rigid rules about men's work (7 A.M. to 7 P.M.) and women's work (raising children full-time), is not much help. Becoming a mother is really an adventure in setting your own goals and your own priorities.

It isn't going to be easy. And your priorities may shift from month to month or from day to day, as your baby's needs, your job demands, and your bank account shifts. But it is really just a matter of setting goals. It is not a matter of "juggling."

Juggling

If you allow others to set your priorities, you will soon be involved in a nonstop juggling act. Some juggling of roles is inevitable for a new mother, but if you watch a group of real jugglers at a fair, you will notice that they juggle for only a few minutes at a time. If they tried to juggle for any substantial length of time (an hour at a stretch, say), they would certainly drop the ball.

Simply juggling roles according to other people's expectations means dropping the ball; it means certain failure. Setting priorities and personal goals is the way to take control of your life.

In interviewing for this book, we were impressed with the number of older mothers who had examined their lives, shifted their goals, and set new and individual priorities. We met Stanford M.B.A.'s who had dropped out of consulting firms and founded their own businesses in order to set their own hours. We met single women who had moved in with other women in order to share child care and expenses. We met women who had hired excellent nannies and continued with their careers. We met women making thoughtful choices, women who were truly able to see themselves as active and effective people in the business of creating their own lives.

MOTHER, HELP THYSELF

The modern mother must create her own life. She must find her balance without constantly looking over her shoulder to see if anyone has caught her doing it wrong. Because if she does look behind her, she will be sure to find an expert there, explaining why she is not perfect, giving advice, blaming the victim. As Ann Dally says in her book *Inventing Motherhood: The Consequences of an Ideal:* "Segregation of children from the world of adult work and leisure has inevitably meant the segregation of their mothers too. . . . One aspect of this segregation is that it greatly increases the mother's exposure to experts [instead of peers and slightly older women] and her dependence upon [them]."

While experts tell the mother that everything in the child's life depends on her actions, they spend very little time actually helping her. When last did you read an article on the subject of how professionals can help mothers relate to their babies? Or suggestions about how society can help a mother who has an "anxiously attached" baby and is clearly not reading the child's signals well? On the other hand, how many covers of magazines at the supermarket checkout counters promise you the secret of running the perfect balancing act?

But even if the experts gave (in the media) the sort of advice they should be giving, something would be missing. How a woman mothers a child depends, among other things, on how she feels about her own life. If she is isolated, lonely, and cut off from her former friends, her ability to mother the child will be affected. When society says, "Go back to work full time at four weeks or forget working," her ability to mother the child is affected. Depressed, unhappy mothers are not good for children.

Few resources are available to help a woman be a productive human being and a mother too. It is as if, for the first time in human history, the two terms were exclusive.

For a moment, in our minds, let us join a group of African (or Fijian or Caribbean) women, some with babies, some without, walking to their yam (or maize or manioc or taro) fields together. Notice how they chat as they work. Notice how the inexperienced mothers get practical help from the old hands. Notice how motherhood has given the new mother status in the group, but not excluded her from it. Notice how nobody is trying to raise a gourmet baby, but merely a reasonably good kid who will be a good worker.

But enough noticing the good parts. Pretty soon, we're going to have to point out how the men have all the status in the village, and how bride-prices and dowries lead to the idea that a woman is basically exchangeable for some cattle. We're going to have to notice weanling diarrhea and possibly mention female infanticide. The third world is definitely not Utopia for women, though actual mothering is often easier there.

Despite the problems in our society, there is also a certain wealth: Adequate food, modern antibiotics, education, and the opportunity to work are available to most people. This richness makes it possible for the older mother to set up her own near-Utopia here. She must be ingenious, she must think about how she will manipulate society in order to get what she needs. But it can be done. You can do it.

A GUIDE TO CREATING YOUR NEAR-UTOPIA

Utopia does not mean dropping out of the work force for years and therefore putting your economic future, your dreams for achievement, and possibly your sanity in jeopardy. It is also not enrolling your baby in day care at four weeks and attempting to return to work as if nothing had happened. In other words, motherhood is not a lifetime career, nor is motherhood just the process of physically recovering from childbirth.

Moreover, becoming a mother does not make you solely and utterly responsible for how your child turns out. The personality and capabilities of your child play a very large role in the outcome, the father plays a large role, and society plays a role—especially in how it supports or inhibits mothering. Recent child-development literature describes the effectiveness of parenting as held by three constraints: 1. the personal resources of the adult; 2. the sources of support and stress in the environment; and 3. the characteristics of the child.

You owe it to your child and yourself to arrange for as few stresses (including economic fear and isolation) and as much support as possible. Having less stress also makes it possible for you to feel warm and loving to your child when you are with her.

We hope that a great deal of your support will come from the baby's father or, for a single mother, from friends and support groups. We will not discuss these personal relationships now because we have done so earlier in the book, but we don't mean to underestimate their importance.

The real problem any working mother faces is arranging society's support. Some reasonable goals follow.

Financial support

Read Chapter 3 again, and set up a childbirth leave. You should be able to arrange to take between four months to a year off work for each baby. This allows you to get to know the baby without strain and worry. It will be lot easier, emotionally, to leave an inquisitive toddler and go off to work than to leave a baby of a few weeks.

Support from other mothers

While you are home with the baby, find other mothers to talk to. Perhaps your Lamaze class can have weekly "bring the baby and have lunch together" reunions. Maybe you can take part in one of the YMCA or YWCA or health club prenatal-postpartum exercise classes. Perhaps you can get involved in La Leche League if you are nursing. It is essential that a new mother not be isolated. You may be able to learn some things about child care from books, but gut-level reassurance is only possible from seeing other mothers and other babies.

Exercise

It is easy to get out of the habit of taking care of yourself. But not taking the time to be healthy is being unfair to yourself and your baby. Many YMCAs, YWCAs, community centers, and health clubs provide child care for a nominal fee while you exercise.

Continue a career or intellectual activity

While you are at home, have some activity that is not related to the baby and is hopefully related to your former or future job. For example, several mothers we interviewed took one course a semester while they were home with their babies. Some took these courses in their chosen field, while others decided that this was a good time to change fields and began to investigate a new area. Or perhaps this is the only period in your life when you will have time to take a course in modern poetry or ancient art.

It is important, emotionally, to have some intellectual involvement that is not baby related. As one mother said, "Having those books there, using my mind, made me feel human. Instead of just getting through the day, I had another goal: finding some time to study. It made all the difference in my attitude."

Examine your own expectations

What are your own beliefs and goals? Do you think, "I can be a perfect mother?" Or, "I can do it all if I just work hard enough?" Be realistic.

Set priorities

Learn to say no. Learn to say, "Not now, maybe later." Deciding what comes first is not a luxury, it is necessary for survival for a new mother. Saying no to other people's requests is your privilege. Your life is your own.

Have fall-back plans

Well, your life isn't completely your own. Babies are time-consuming, and the time they consume is not well scheduled. Some mornings you won't have had a good night's sleep. One day the day-care center is sure to call you while you are in an important meeting to tell you that your child has an earache. It becomes important to remember that few things in the work world or the home world are really and truly time-critical on an hourly basis. By staying flexible, you can rethink your plans and make a contingency arrangement in almost every circumstance, so long as you can avoid getting deeply upset at having to take a more roundabout path to a goal. This is especially true for your work life. Your son's earache hurts *now,* but there will probably be another meeting in a week.

Arrange part-time work

Sometime between when the baby is four months and a year old, you probably will want to go back to work part time. Can you arrange this? You might want to read the books *Working from Home* or *Of Cradles and Careers* (see Chapter References) for ideas.

Often, however, after the first months, full-time work becomes a financial necessity. There is no need to feel guilty about this, even if you would have preferred to stay home longer. You've taken the time to give your baby a good start. You thought enough about his development to play with him and talk to him through those early days.

When do we recommend going back to work full time? The first question is: What is full time?

For some women, full time is seventy hours a week on the job. These women, once they become mothers, can't really go back to work "full time" at all, unless they are willing to hire a nanny. Hopefully, they are paid well enough to afford adequate help. As one mother, a physician, says, "How do I spend time with my children? Simple. They are my first priority, after working. Which also means that I don't cook, I don't clean, and I don't go grocery shopping. We've had the same woman living with us for years, and she runs the household." If you work significantly more than forty hours a week, this is the arrangement that makes it possible.

What if full time is "just full time," forty hours a week? In Utopia, no family would have both parents involved in jobs with rigid schedules. If she worked forty hours a week, he would be self-employed or a student, with more time flexibility. If he worked forty hours, she would freelance. But we're designing near-Utopia here, and in near-Utopia it is probably best to wait for a year before going back full time—or perhaps even longer. Leaving a three-year-old full time is easier than leaving a one-year-old. But such waits aren't strictly necessary. It all depends on your finances, the stability of the part-time arrangement you made earlier, your child-care arrangements, the personality of your child, and your own desires.

A FINAL WORD

To be both effective mothers and effective and self-supporting adults in this society, women have to be ingenious. They have to reject the either-or concepts of mother or career woman. They have to reject the either-or concepts of back full time at four weeks or forget your career. They have to reject the overwhelming guilt and isolation that society visits upon mothers.

In place of these rejected beliefs, women must substitute the idea of *time out* for motherhood: Motherhood as an interruption of a career, not an end to it. Motherhood as an enricher of life, not the end to adult behavior. Motherhood as an enhancer of life, not a guilt producer.

In interviewing women for this book, we were delighted and affirmed to see how many over-thirty mothers had challenged society's negatives and come up with their own positives. How many had managed to take time out ("It was important to me") and afterwards were back at work, living full and exciting lives. Stressful lives, yes, but the stress was worth something. As Dr. Hans Selye, the founder of modern stress research, put it: "To be without stress entirely is to be dead." There is joy in working hard toward your own goals.

Some people in this society wear literal and figurative sweatshirts that say HE WHO DIES WITH THE MOST TOYS, WINS. The over-thirty mother is not wearing that slogan; she has chosen a child, despite her adult knowledge that a child is far more expensive than a BMW, a VCR, and two trips to Europe put together.

In short, the over-thirty mother is capable of close to the ultimate in truly adult living: knowing and setting her own priorities. Loving and working.

And her children will reflect this.

To all the women we interviewed for this book: We're glad we met you. You've helped us appreciate the ingenuity, wisdom, and nurturance of over-thirty mothers. Without you, of course, there would be no book. But without having learned who you are and how you've done things, there would certainly be no upbeat ending.

R E F E R E N C E S

Note: Some of the chapter references are described more fully in the annotated bibliography.

Chapter 1

Baldwin, Wendy, and Christine Winquist Nord. "Delayed Childbearing in the U.S.: Facts and Fictions." *Population Bulletin* (Population Reference Bureau, Washington, D.C.) 39, no. 4 (1984).

Daniels, Pamela, and Kathy Weingarten. *Sooner or Later: The Timing of Parenthood in Adult Lives.* New York: W. W. Norton, 1982.

Feldman, S. Shirley. "Predicting Strain in Mothers and Fathers of 6-Month-Old Infants: A Short-term Longitudinal Study." To appear in *Men's Transitions to Parenthood,* edited by P. Berman and F. Pedersen. Hillsdale, N.J.: Lawrence Erlbaum, 1987 (book in preparation).

Feldman, S. Shirley, and Sharon C. Nash. "Antecedents of Early Parenting." To appear in *Origins of Nurturance,* edited by Fogel and Melson. Hillsdale, N.J.: Lawrence Erlbaum, 1986.

Friedan, Betty. *The Feminine Mystique.* New York: W. W. Norton, 1974 (first published 1964).

Friedan, Betty. *The Second Stage.* New York: Simon & Schuster, 1971.

Gelb, Joyce, and Marian Lief Palley. *Women and Public Policies.* Princeton, N.J.: Princeton University Press, 1982.

Greer, Germaine. *The Female Eunuch.* New York: McGraw-Hill, 1971.

———, *Sex and Destiny: The Politics of Human Fertility.* New York: Harper & Row, 1984.

Hoffreth, Sandra. "Long-Term Economic Consequences for Women of Delayed Childbearing and Reduced Family Size." *Demography* 21, no. 2 (1984): 141.

National Association of Realtors. "Affordability Index." Washington, D.C.: National Association of Realtors, 1984.

Ragozin, Arlene S., et al. "The Effects of Maternal Age on Parenting Role." *Developmental Psychology* 18 (1982): 627–634.

Chapter 2

Cohen, Wayne, et al. "Risk of Labor Abnormalities with Advancing Maternal Age." *Obstetrics and Gynecology* 55, no. 4 (1984): 414ff.

Cruikshank, Dwight P., et al. "Midtrimester Amniocentesis: Analysis of 923 Cases with Neonatal Follow-Up." *American Journal of Obstetrics and Gynecology* 146, no. 2 (1983): 204ff.

Discover. "Alternative to Amniocentesis." May 1985.

Dobhzansky, Theodosius. *Mankind Evolving.* New Haven: Yale University Press, 1962.

"Fetal Alcohol Syndrome: Public Awareness Week." *Center for Disease Control Weekly Report.* Atlanta, Ga.: 13 January 1984.

Good, Erica. "Early Test for Birth Defects Tried at UCSF." *San Francisco Chronicle,* 29 March 1985.

Hingson, Ralph, et al. "Effects of Maternal Drinking and Marijuana Use on Fetal Growth and Development." *Pediatrics* 70 (October 1982): 539 ff.

Jefferson Medical College. *Bulletin on First Trimester Fetal Genetic Diagnosis.* Philadelphia: Thomas Jefferson University.

Kitzinger, Sheila. *Birth Over Thirty.* New York: Viking, 1985.

Kruse, Jerry. "Alcohol Use During Pregnancy." *American Family Physician,* April 1984.

McCauley, Carole Spearin. *Pregnancy after 35.* New York: Pocket Books, 1976.

McIntosh, Ian. "Smoking and Pregnancy: Attributable Risks and Public Health Implications." *Canadian Journal of Public Health* 75 (1984): 141.

Menken, Jane, and Ulla Larsen. "Age and Fecundity: How Late Can You Wait?" Article submitted for publication and quoted in Baldwin, W., and Christine Winquist Nord, "Delayed Childbearing the the U. S.: Facts and Fictions." *Population Bulletin* (Population Reference Bureau, Washington, D.C.) 39, no.4 (1984).

Naeye, Richard L. "Maternal Age, Obstetric Complications, and the Outcome of Pregnancy." *Obstetrics and Gynecology* 61, no.2 (1983): 210ff.

Niaza, Meena, et al. "Trophoblastic Sampling in Early Pregnancy: Culture of Rapidly Dividing Cells from Immature Placental Villi." *British Journal of Obstetrics and Gynecology* 88 (1981): 1081ff.

Rubin, Sylvia P. *It's Not Too Late for a Baby: For Women and Men over Thirty-five.* Englewood Cliffs, N.J.: Prentice-Hall, 1980.

Rubin, S.P., et al. "Genetic Counseling Before Prenatal Diagnosis for Advanced Maternal Age: An Important Medical Safeguard." *Obstetrics and Gynecology* 62, no.2 (1983).

Shepard, Thomas, M.D. *Catalogue of Teratogenic Agents.* Baltimore, Md.: Johns Hopkins Press, 1983.

Chapter 3

Anderson, Judith. "What It Costs to Rear a Child." *San Francisco Chronicle,* 9 March 1982.

Bundy, Darcie. *The Affordable Baby.* New York: Harper & Row, 1985.

Edwards, Carolyn. "The Cost of Raising a Child." *American Demographics* 3 (July–August 1981): 25–29.

Lesko, Wendy and Matthew. *Maternity Sourcebook.* New York: Warner Books, 1984.

Chapter 4

Duncan, Barbara. *The Single Mother's Survival Manual,* 1984. R & E Publishers, P.O. Box 2008, Saratoga, Ca. 95070.

Greywolf, Elizabeth S. *The Single Mother's Handbook.* New York: Quill Press, 1984.

Joseph, Nadine. "Jewish Women Find Alternatives to Daddy." *Northern California Jewish Bulletin,* 17 May 1985.

Lee, Deborah. *Self-Help for Single Mothers: A Model Peer-Supported Program,* 1984. Available through the Early Single Parenting Project, 1005 Market Street, #313, San Francisco, Ca. 94103.

Mack, Phyllis. "Choosing Single Motherhood." *Ms.* magazine, November 1984.

National Commission on Working Women. *Working Mothers and Their Families: A Fact Sheet.* Washington, D.C., 1984.

Oakland Feminist Women's Health Center, 2930 McClure Street, Oakland, Ca. 94609. (For information on donor insemination.)

Chapter 5

Cath, Stanley H., Alan Gurwitt, and John Munder Ross, eds. *Father and Child: Development and Clinical Perspectives.* Boston: Little, Brown, 1982. Articles used:

"Engrossment: The Newborn's Impact on the Father," by Martin Greenberg and Norman Morris.

"Observation on the Father-Infant Relationship," by Michael W. Yogman.

"A Note on the Father's Contribution to the Daughter's Ways of Loving and Working," by Lora Heims Tessman.

"Patterns of Expectant Fatherhood: A Study of the Fathers of a Group of Premature Infants," by James A. Herzog.

Colman, Arthur. *Earth Father Sky Father: The Changing Concept of Fathering.* Englewood Cliffs, N.J.: Prentice-Hall, 1981.

Cordes, Colleen. "Researchers Make Room for Father." *American Psychological Association Monitor,* December 1983.

Erikson, Erik H. *Childhood and Society.* New York: W. W. Norton, 1963.

Feldman, S. Shirley, Sharon Churnin Nash, and Barbara G. Aschenbrenner. "Antecedents of Fathering." *Child Development* 54 (1983): 1628–1636.

Heinowitz, Jack. *Pregnant Fathers: How Fathers Can Enjoy and Share the Experiences of Pregnancy and Childbirth.* Englewood Cliffs, N.J.: Prentice-Hall, 1982.

Lamb, Michael, ed. *The Role of the Father in Child Development* (part of the Wiley series on personality processes). New York: John Wiley, 1981. Articles used:

"Fathers and Child Development: An Integrative Overview," by Michael Lamb.

"The Role of the Father: An Anthropological Perspective," by Mary Maxwell Katz and Melvin J. Konner.

"Father Influences Viewed in a Family Context," by Frank A. Pedersen.

"The Father and Sex Role Development," by Henry B. Biller.

"The Development of Father-Infant Relations," by Michael Lamb.

Lewis, Joy S. "Some Fathers-to-Be Suffer Symptoms of Wives' Pregnancies." *San Jose Mercury,* 4 April 1985.

Stephen, Beverly. "Time Off for New Fathers." *San Francisco Chronicle,* 17 September 1984.

Chapter 6

Daniels, Pamela, and Kathy Weingarten. *Sooner or Later: The Timing of Parenthood in Adult Lives.* New York: W. W. Norton, 1982.

Feldman, Silvia. *Making up Your Mind about Motherhood: The Complete Guide for Making the Most Important Decision of Your Life.* New York: Bantam, 1985.

Scott, Lucy. *Parenthood After Thirty Resource Manual,* 1981. Available through Parenthood After Thirty, 451 Vermont, Berkeley, Ca. 94707.

Sheehy, Gail. *Passages.* New York: E. P. Dutton, 1974.

Chapter 7

Chesler, Phyllis. *With Child: A Diary of Motherhood.* New York: Thomas Crowell, 1979.

Goldberg, Susan. "Parent-Infant Bonding: Another Look." *Child Development* 54 (1983): 1355–1382.

Gordon, Pippa. "Childbirth after 35: The Tough Choices." *San Francisco Bay Area Guardian,* 15 February 1984.

Karmel, Marjorie. *Thank You, Dr. Lamaze.* New York: Doubleday, 1959.

Oakley, Ann. *Becoming a Mother.* New York: Schocken Books, 1979.

Rapp, Rayna. "The Ethics of Choice." *Ms.* magazine, April 1984.

Stautberg, Susan Schiffer. *Pregnancy Nine to Five: The Career Woman's Guide to Pregnancy and Motherhood.* New York: Simon & Schuster, 1985.

Chapter 8

Asimov, Isaac. *In Joy Still Felt: The Autobiography of Isaac Asimov, 1954–1978.* New York: Doubleday, 1980.

Brazelton, T. Berry. *Infants and Mothers: Differences in Development.* New York: Dell, 1969.

Eheart, Brenda Krause, and Susan Martel. *The Fourth Trimester: On Becoming a Mother.* Norwalk, Ct.: Appleton-Century Crofts, 1983.

Feldman, S. Shirley, and Sharon C. Nash. "Antecedents of Early Parenting." To appear in *Origins of Nurturance,* edited by Fogel and Melson. Hillsdale, N.J.: Lawrence Erlbaum, 1986.

La Leche League International. 9616 Minneapolis Avenue, Franklin Park, Illinois 60131.

LaRossa, Ralph and Maureen Mulligan. *Transition to Parenthood: How Infants Change Families.* Beverly Hills, Ca.: Sage Library of Social Research, 1981.

Miller, Warren B., and Lucile F. Newman, eds. *The First Child and Family Formation.* Chapel Hill: University of North Carolina, Carolina Population Center, 1978.

Oakley, Ann. *Becoming a Mother.* New York: Schocken Books, 1979.

Pryor, Karen. *Nursing Your Baby.* New York: Pocket Books, 1974.

Raphael, Dana. *The Tender Gift: Breastfeeding.* Englewood Cliffs, N.J.: Prentice-Hall, 1973.

Scarr, Sandra. *Mother Care, Other Care.* New York: Basic Books, 1984.

Staurberg, Susan Schippe. *Pregnancy Nine to Five: The Career Woman's Guide to Pregnancy and Motherhood.* New York, Simon and Schuster, 1985.

Thompson, Richard. "Mystery of Crib Death." *FDA Consumer Magazine.* April 1983.

White, Burton. *The First Three Years of Life.* New York: Avon, 1975.

Winter, Sara K. "Fantasies at Breastfeeding Time." *Psychology Today* 3, no. 8 (January 1970): 30.

Chapter 9

Baldwin, Wendy, and Christine Winquist Nord. "Delayed Childbearing in the U.S.: Facts and Fictions." *Population Bulletin* (Population Reference Bureau, Washington, D.C.) 39, no. 4 (1984).

"Behind Hiring of More Temporary Employees." *U.S. News and World Report,* 25 February 1985.

Edwards, Paul and Sarah. *Working from Home: Everything You Need to Know about Living and Working under the Same Roof.* Los Angeles: Jeremy P. Tarcher, 1985.

Lowman, Kay. *Of Cradles and Careers: A Guide to Reshaping Your Job to Include a Baby in Your Life.* Franklin Park, Ill.: La Leche League International, 1984.

Shreve, Anita. "Careers and the Lure of Motherhood." *New York Times Magazine,* 21 November 1982.

―――. "The Maternity Backlash: Women vs. Women." *Working Woman,* March 1985.

Toman, Barbara. "Maternity Costs, Parenthood and Career Overtax Some Women, Despite Best Intentions." *Wall Street Journal,* 7 September 1983.

"Where Poor People Are Better Off." *San Francisco Chronicle,* 26 January 1984.

Women's Bureau. "A Working Woman's Guide to Her Job Rights." Washington, D.C.: U.S. Department of Labor, January 1984 (Leaflet 55).

————. "Twenty Facts on Women Workers." Washington, D.C.: U. S. Department of Labor, 1982.

Organizations specializing in part-time work guidance (newsletters, brochures, support groups):

New Ways to Work
149 Ninth St.
San Francisco, Ca. 94103

Catalyst
14 East 60th St.
New York, N.Y. 10022

Chapter 10

Staff of Bananas Child Care Information and Referral Service for families in Alameda County, California. *Bananas Guide for Parents and Children.* Berkeley, Ca.: Wingbaum Press, 1982.

Brazelton, T. Berry. *Working and Caring.* New York: Merloyd Lawrence, 1985.

Clarke-Stewart, Alison. *Daycare.* The Developing Child Series. Cambridge, Mass.: Harvard University Press, 1982.

Fooner, Andrea. "Six Good Solutions for Childcare." *Working Woman* (October 1985): 173.

Gave, Keith. "Don't Call Them Baby Sitters: New Nanny School Wants to Make Child Care a Profession." *San Francisco Chronicle,* 21 April 1983.

Ricks, Thomas E. "Researchers Say Day-Care Centers Implicated in Spread of Disease." *Wall Street Journal,* 5 September 1985.

Scarr, Sandra. *Mother Care, Other Care.* New York: Basic Books, 1984.

Siegal-Gorelich, Bryna. *The Working Parents' Guide to Child Care.* Boston: Little, Brown, 1983.

Walsh, Mary Williams. "Career Women Rely on Day Care, Nannies to Meet Child-Care Needs." *Wall Street Journal,* 25 September 1984.

Chapter 11

Braiker, Harriet B. "How to Handle the Back-to-Stress Season." *Working Woman,* September 1985.

Caplan, Paula J., and Ian Hall-McCorquode. "Mother Blaming in Major Clinical Journals." *American Journal of Orthopsychiatry* (July 1985): 345–365.

Dally, Ann. *Inventing Motherhood: The Consequences of an Ideal.* New York: Schocken Books, 1983.

Goodman, Ellen. *At Large.* New York: Simon & Schuster, 1981.

Kirsch, Jonathan. "Gourmet Babies." *California,* January 1983.

Progrebin, Letty Cottin. *Growing Up Free: Raising Your Child in the 80's.* New York: Bantam Books, 1981.

Ricks, Thomas E. "New Minority of Mothers at Home Find Support in Family Centers." *Wall Street Journal,* 25 October 1985.

Sears, William, M.D. *Creative Parenting.* New York: Dodd, Mead, 1983.

Alphafetoprotein

A protein produced by the developing fetus and excreted into the amniotic ·fluid. An elevated AFP level in pregnancy is a sign of fetal distress, especially major neural-tube birth defects or impending abortion or premature birth.

Amniocentesis

The removal of a small amount of amniotic fluid by the use of a hollow needle placed through the abdomen and into the uterus.

Amniotic fluid

The fluid that surrounds the developing fetus contained within the amniotic membranes. This fluid acts as a protective mechanism for the fetus and can be used for diagnosing certain fetal abnormalities, fetal maturity, and placental function.

Attachment

A process by which a child forms an affectional tie with the mother or other main caretaker and devotes powerful energy to retaining visual and auditory contact with her, shows emotional distress at separation, and joy at reunion.

Birth defects

Any physical or mental abnormalities present at birth; they may be of genetic or environmental origin.

Carrier (genetic)

A person who carries a genetic characteristic as part of his or her chromosomes. The characteristic may have no observable manifestations but can be passed on to the next generation.

Cervix

Lower part of the uterus (mouth), which extends into the vagina and connects the vagina and cavity of the uterus via its central opening.

Cesarean section

The birth of a baby through the abdomen by surgical incisions into the abdominal and uterine walls.

Chorionic villi biopsy

Removal of a small portion of tissue from the surface of the chorion (a precursor of the placenta) for diagnostic assessment. The procedure is performed at approximately the eighth week of pregnancy by insertion of a catheter into the uterus through the vagina.

Chromosomes

Microscopic units located within the nucleus of every cell which contain the basic hereditary factors in the form of genes. There are 46 chromosomes in every cell except the reproductive cells (egg and sperm cells), which contain 23.

Colostrum

A thick, yellowish fluid, which is the first liquid obtained from the breast by the newborn.

Conception

The uniting of the male and female reproductive cells (sperm and egg) resulting in the beginning of pregnancy (fertilization).

Diabetes

An abnormality in the body's ability to produce insulin and, therefore, to process sugars. Age at onset and severity have both genetic and environmental components.

Donor insemination

A procedure in which live sperm from a donor are placed by syringe at the entrance to the cervix at the time of ovulation in the menstrual cycle.

Down's syndrome

Also called mongolism or trisomy 21. A chromosome abnormality involving the presence of an extra chromosome (47 in all), usually present in all cells of the body; there are three #21 chromosomes instead of the normal two. Many associated physical abnormalities can be present in addition to mental retardation. Occurrence increases with advanced maternal age.

Eclampsia

Convulsions and coma occurring in a pregnant woman or soon after birth. It is generally associated with hypertension, edema, and/or proteinuria and can usually be prevented with close obstetrical care.

Ectopic pregnancy

Abnormal implantation or attachment of the embryo outside the uterus. The most common site is within a fallopian tube (tubal pregnancy), but implantation can occur elsewhere in the abdomen.

Endometriosis

The presence of endometrial tissue (tissue that normally lines the interior of the uterus) elsewhere in the abdomen. The tissue can adhere to and block normal functioning of other organs, such as the ovaries and fallopian tubes, causing infertility.

Episiotomy

An incision or surgical cut in the perineum performed to widen the opening of the vagina to ease passage of the baby's head during childbirth.

Fallopian tubes

The portions of the female reproductive system through which an egg passes en route from the ovary (where it is formed) to the uterus (where implantation normally occurs).

Fetal alcohol syndrome

A combination of birth defects that are characteristic of some infants born to mothers who have a history of heavy alcohol use.

Fibroids

Benign growths in the uterus that are composed of fibrous and muscle tissue; they occur more frequently in older women.

Genital herpes

A viral disease characterized by blisters on the genitalia. Herpes virus present in a woman's birth canal can be picked up by her infant during labor and delivery.

Huntington's chorea

A rare hereditary disease characterized by chronic progressive chorea and mental deterioration, terminating in dementia.

Hypertension

A sustained elevated blood pressure.

Lactation

The secretion of milk.

Menarche

First occurrence of the menstrual discharge.

Menopause

Cessation of the menstrual cycle.

Moro's reflex

An infant suddenly throws its arms out in response to being startled.

Neural tube defects

Malformations resulting from an abnormal development in the neural tube. The neural tube is the embryonic structure that will become part of the spine. Spina bifida (below) is one of the most common neural tube defects.

Oxytocin

The hormone that stimulates contraction of the uterine muscles.

Placenta

A spongy structure implanted in the uterine wall during a pregnancy. It supplies vital oxygen and nutrients to the fetus and removes waste products via the umbilical cord.

After delivery the placenta is expelled (also called the afterbirth).

Placenta previa

A condition in which the placenta is located in the lower portion of the uterine wall so that it partially or completely covers the cervical opening.

Primigravida

A woman pregnant for the first time (regardless of age).

Progesterone

The hormone whose function it is to prepare the uterus for the reception and development of the fertilized ovum.

Prolactin

The hormone that stimulates and sustains lactation.

Sickle cell disease

A hereditary condition characterized by sickle-shaped red blood cells and impaired red-blood-cell function.

Spina bifida

A defect in the spinal column that occurs as early as four weeks' gestation. It can be a closed or an open defect, which can be totally asymtomatic or else more severe, involving the spinal cord.

Strange-situation test

A controlled laboratory situation, designed by Ainsworth, in which babies are observed in an unfamiliar environment with their mother alternately present and absent. The baby's behavior toward a stranger is observed with the mother present and absent.

Syndrome

A group of symptoms or characteristics which by themselves may not be significant but when occurring together can form the basis for a specific diagnosis.

Tay-sachs disease

A hereditary deficiency in the essential enzyme hexosaminidase A, leading to neurological deterioration and death of affected infants early in life.

Thalassemia

A heterogeneous group of hereditary anemias observed originally in persons of Mediterranean heritage.

Trimester

A time period in pregnancy involving three months. There are three trimesters: The first (months one to three), the second (months four to six), and the third (months seven to nine).

Ultrasound

A noninvasive diagnostic test based on high-frequency sound waves that are transmitted through a transducer via a fluid. An image is reproduced on a screen and photographed for diagnostic purposes.

B I B L I O G R A P H Y

Suggested books for further reading are offered here on specific subjects. They are arranged to follow the topics in the book.

Part One: The Decision

Friedan, Betty. *The Second Stage.* New York: Simon & Schuster, 1971. An excellent book on where women are today and the directions in which feminism should evolve.

Daniels, Pamela, and Kathy Weingarten. *Sooner or Later: The Timing of Parenthood in Adult Lives.* New York: W.W. Norton, 1982. A good book about how life works for "early-sequence" and "late-sequence" parents. Some jargon.

Rubin, Sylvia P. *It's Not Too Late for a Baby: For Women and Men Over Thirty-five.* Prentice-Hall, 1980. All the information you ever needed (and more) on statistics of birth defects and complications of pregnancy. A little frightening, in the same way medical texts are frightening: So many potential problems! Somewhat out of date on chorionic villi sampling, however.

McCauley, Carole Spearin. *Pregnancy after 35.* New York: Pocket Books, 1976. More general than Rubin's book: fewer statistics; easier to read; more about the experience of pregnancy.

Kitzinger, Sheila. *Birth over Thirty.* New York: Viking, 1985. How to manage your own pregnancy, avoid being pushed around by doctors and the medical establishment, and have a natural birth. Good advice; just take it with a grain of salt.

Lesko, Wendy and Matthew. *Maternity Sourcebook.* New York: Warner Books, 1984. Lists of things to buy and how to buy them; advantages and disadvantages of various childbirth preparation methods.

Bundy, Darcie. *The Affordable Baby.* New York: Harper & Row, 1985. Good advice on medical insurance and how to choose baby equipment. Nothing on planning for your leave, though.

Greywolf, Elizabeth S. *The Single Mother's Handbook.* New York: Quill Press, 1984. Much useful advice, though a good deal of it aimed at divorced women with older children.

Lee, Deborah. *Self-Help for Single Mothers: A Model Peer-Supported Program,* 1984. Available through the Early Single Parenting Project, 1005 Market Street, #313, San Francisco, Ca. 94103. How to set up a support group. Mostly for professionals (social workers, psychologists) but interesting for mothers, also.

Duncan, Barbara. *The Single Mother's Survival Manual,* 1984. R & E Publishers, P.O. Box 2008, Saratoga, Ca. 95070. Lots of good advice, from dating to job rights.

Colman, Arthur. *Earth Father Sky Father: The Changing Concept of Fathering.* Englewood Cliffs, N.J.: Prentice-Hall, 1981. An interesting conceptual approach: The "earth father" is more involved in nurturing; the "sky father" is concerned with inspiring and providing.

Heinowitz, Jack. *Pregnant Fathers: How Fathers Can Enjoy and Share the Experiences of Pregnancy and Childbirth.* Englewood Cliffs, N.J.: Prentice-Hall, 1982. Interesting advice and anecdotes about having a pregnant wife. Not really about fathering.

Scott, Lucy. *Parenthood After Thirty Resource Manual.* 1981. Available through Parenthood After Thirty, 451 Vermont, Berkeley, Ca. 94707. A guide to the decision itself. Used in workshops and training sessions.

Feldman, Silvia. *Making up Your Mind about Motherhood: The Complete Guide for Making the Most Important Decision of Your Life.* New York: Bantam, 1985. Good sections on adoption and on the handicapped mother.

Part 2: Pregnancy and Beyond

Stautberg, Susan Schiffer. *Pregnancy Nine to Five: The Career Woman's Guide to Pregnancy and Motherhood.* New York: Simon & Schuster, 1985. Mostly about negotiating your leave and going back to the office. Tends to use examples of very well paid women, in glamorous careers. Nevertheless, good advice about things to consider for the negotiation-with-your-boss process, and for staying in touch with the office when you are first home with the baby.

Brazelton, T. Berry. *Infants and Mothers: Differences in Development.* New York: Dell, 1969. Through the day and through the months in three families, one with a quiet baby, one with an average baby, one with an active baby. Overall, reassuring.

White, Burton. *The First Three Years of Life.* New York: Avon, 1975. A little dry, but lots of useful and interesting information on infant development.

Pryor, Karen. *Nursing Your Baby.* New York: Pocket Books, 1974. Helpful hints and scientific explanations from a mother who is also a biologist.

Eheart, Brenda Krause, and Susan Martel. *The Fourth Trimester: On Becoming a Mother.* Norwalk, Ct.: Appleton-Century Crofts, 1983. A guide to the predictable maternal emotions of the first few weeks and how to help yourself cope.

Edwards, Paul and Sarah. *Working from Home: Everything You Need to Know about Living and Working under the Same Roof.* Los Angeles: Jeremy P. Tarcher, 1985. Possible jobs, exploring whether you want to be an employee or self-employed, how to organize your life, even how to avoid getting fat from being so close to the refrigerator!

Lowman, Kaye. *Of Cradles and Careers: A Guide to Reshaping Your Job to Include a Baby in Your Life.* Franklin Park, Ill.: La Leche League International, 1984. Case studies of ingenious women. Many ideas, such as how to persuade your employer to give you a reduced work week.

Clarke-Stewart, Alison. *Daycare.* The Developing Child Series. Cambridge, Mass.: Harvard University Press, 1982. A thoughtful book, but concentrates on the older child.

Siegal-Gorelich, Bryna. *The Working Parents' Guide to Child Care.* Boston: Little, Brown, 1983. Day care from infancy to preschool. Lots of examples and guidelines.

Scarr, Sandra. *Mother Care, Other Care.* New York: Basic Books, 1984. Philosophical. A strong argument that well-chosen day care doesn't hurt children. Comments on how society views working and stay-at-home mothers.

Brazelton, T. Berry. *Working and Caring.* New York: Merloyd Lawrence, 1985. Through the day in three working families. How to deal with morning and evening stress.

Goodman, Ellen. *At Large.* New York: Simon & Schuster, 1981. A series of interesting and enlightening essays on motherhood, working, and life in general.

Dally, Ann. *Inventing Motherhood: The Consequences of an Ideal.* New York: Schocken Books, 1983. A fascinating book: historical perspective on mothering, what it is, and who should do it.

ABOUT THE AUTHORS

Dr. Lucy Scott, a psychologist and educator, is currently the supervisor of Parent's Place, and the former director of the Parenthood After Thirty project. She teaches, lectures, and presents workshops throughout the country. Dr. Scott has a clinical practice in Berkeley, California, and teaches at the University of San Francisco. She has two daughters, Cynthia and Susan, in their thirties.

Meredith Angwin is a scientist, a mother, a wife, and a writer. She holds a Master's degree in physical chemistry, and is a project manager at the Electric Power Research Institute in Palo Alto, California. She has three patents to her credit and several technical articles. She also writes poetry, and is now a columnist for *Frequent Flyer* magazine. Ms. Angwin lives in Palo Alto with her husband, George, and their teenaged children, Julia and Ilan.